FOOT   Acupuncture

CLINICAL TREATMENT

足临床疗法

Sumiko Knudsen

Ph.D
Practitioner. DK

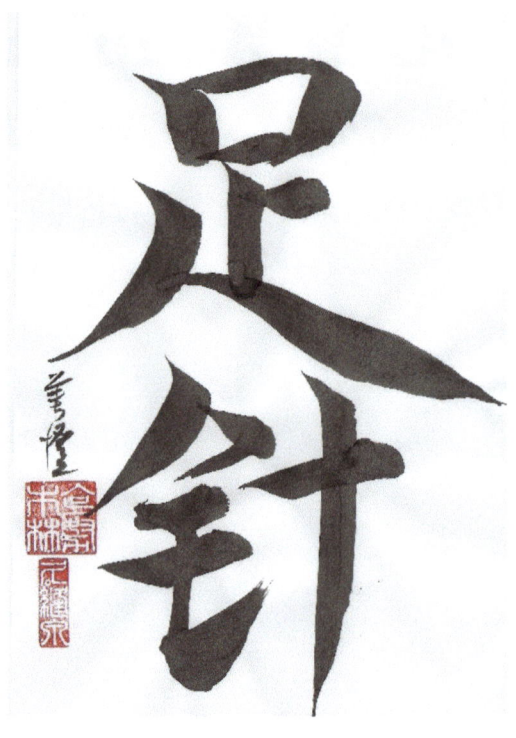

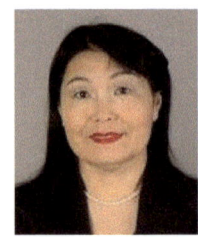

Sumiko Knudsen was born in Japan, and she has lived in USA, UK and Denmark for many years. She graduated at Nordic College of Chinese Acupuncture in Denmark, and then she went on and studied at Beijing University of TCM in China. After that she studied and graduated at Nanjing University of TCM in China. and she earned Ph.D. She is a private practitioner in Denmark.

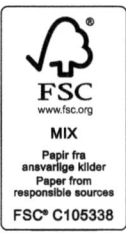

© 2022 Sumiko Knudsen
Forlag: BoD – Books on Demand, Hellerup, Danmark
Tryk: BoD – Books on Demand, Norderstedt, Tyskland

ISBN: 9788743047322

CONTENTS

10

INTRODUCTION

In acupuncture, the foot is a projection of the body.

The foot has correspondence with the organs of the body. The reflecting areas of internal organs are on the sole of the foot, and the foot areas have correspondence to the organs of the body.

Foot Acupuncture therapy for the treatment of diseases is a therapeutic method applying different types of stimulation at various specific parts of the foot to promote circulation of Qi and Blood through meridians.

The foot can be used to diagnose and treat diseases as the foot is closely connected with other parts of the body in a common internal environment.

Foot therapy originated much earlier than other therapies according to the history of Chinese Traditional Medicine.

Foot therapy is safe, reliable, effective, and easy to perform for both early diagnosis and treatment of many diseases. Foot therapy is non-medicinal nature and can relieves pain.

Therefore, it has attracted the attention of more people in the world.

Sumiko Knudsen 克努森澄子

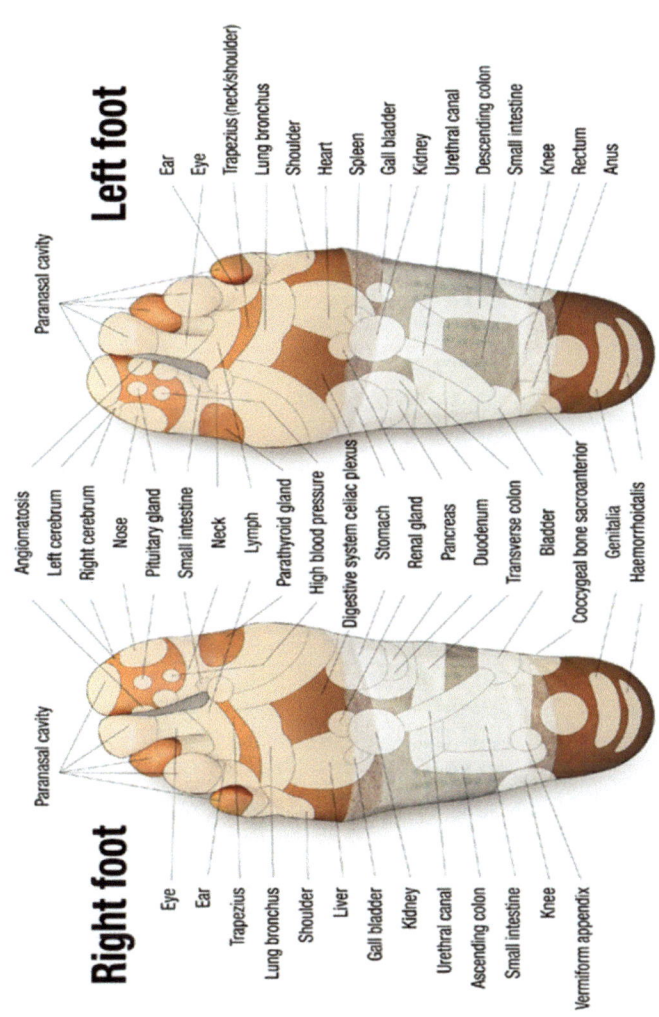

Foot point

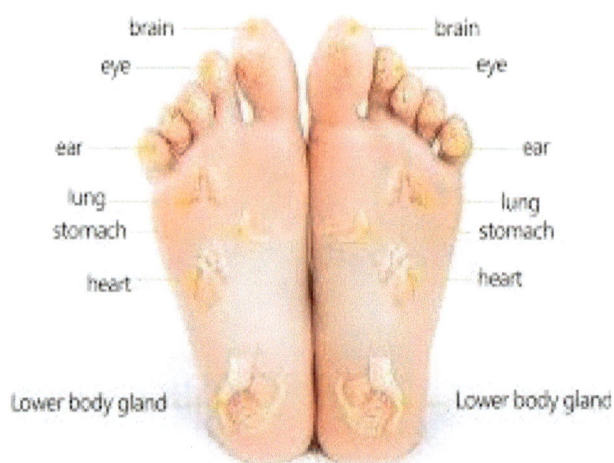

Human's organ

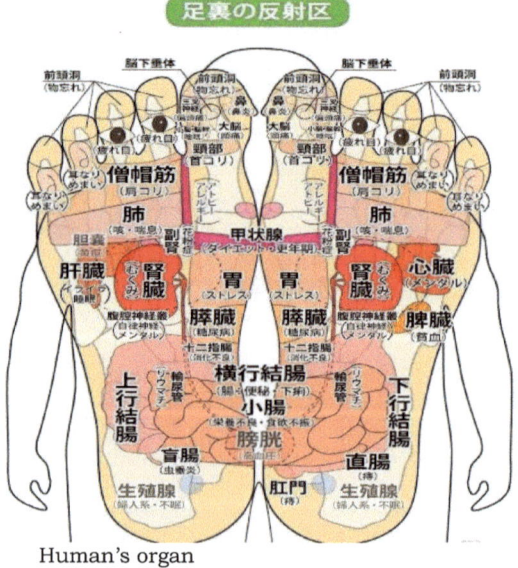

Human's organ

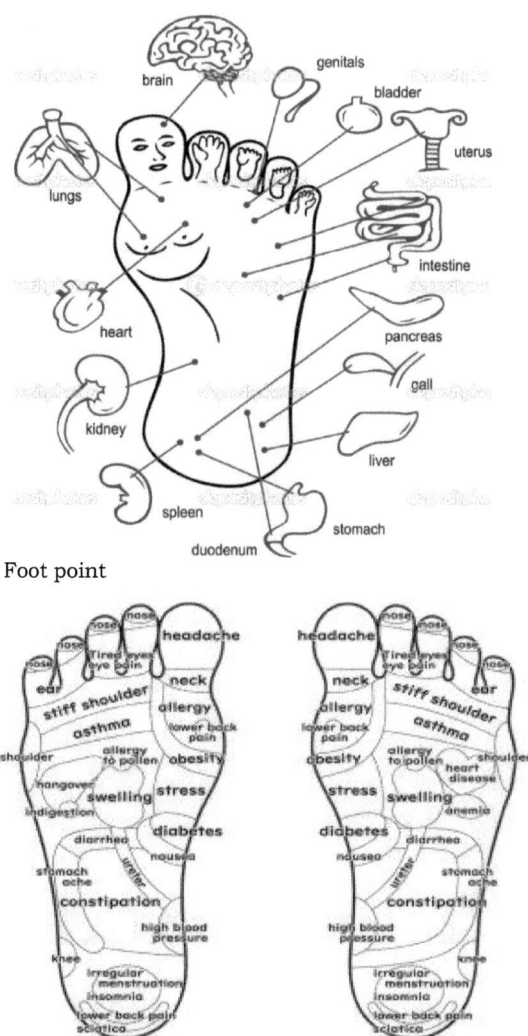

Foot point

Common disease

Chapter 1. Foot Therapy

Foot therapy originated much earlier than other therapies according to the history of Chinese Traditional Medicine. The pain caused by disease could be relieved by applying some stimulation to the area of the foot by hands or acupuncture or others.

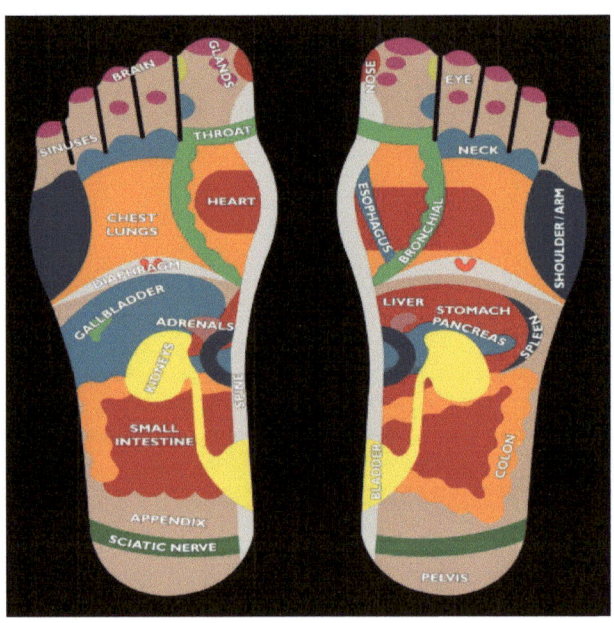

I. Reflecting Areas of Internal Organ

Foot areas correspond to the organs of the body. The big toe corresponds to the head of brain and proximal end of the big toe corresponds to the neck.

The reflecting areas of organs on the left side of the body correspond to the left foot. The right side of the body corresponds to the right foot. Organs such as Kidney, Lung and Ureter in pairs have corresponding areas on both feet. The organs on the midline, such as the cerebrum, cerebellum, nose, tonsils, stomach, and spinal column have the medial borders of both feet. Liver, spleen, and ears are the lateral borders of both feet.

The projected areas of the cerebrum, frontal sinus, trigeminal nerves, eyes, and ears are on the contralateral foot.

Projected area of the trigeminal nerve on the left foot is to treat on the right of the face, and on the right foot is to treat on the left of the face.

1. Right sole: Diagram of reflecting areas

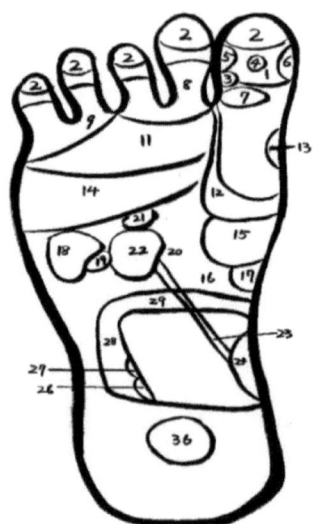

Fig. 1 Reflecting areas on Sole of right foot

1. Head (brain), left hemisphere
2. Left frontal sinus

7. Nose
8. Neck
9. Left eye
10. Left ear

3. Brain stem and cerebellum
4. Pituitary gland
5. Left trigeminal
6. nerve
11. trapezius muscle (neck, shoulder)
12. thyroid gland
13. parathyroid gland

14. lung and bronchus
15. stomach
16. duodenum
17. pancreas
18. liver
19. gallbladder
20. celiac plexus
21. adrenal gland
22. kidney
23. ureter
24. urinary bladder

26. cecum (appendix)
27. ileocecal valve
28. ascending colon
29. transverse colon
36. reproductive gland (ovary or testis)

2. Left sole: Diagram of reflecting areas

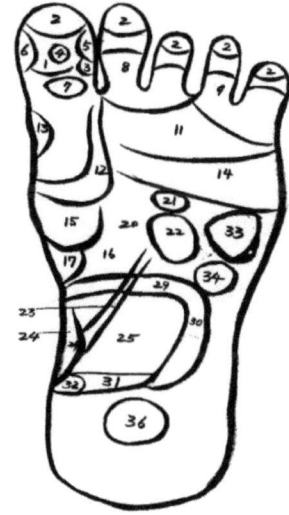

Fig. 2 Reflecting areas on Sole of left foot

1. Head (brain), right hemisphere
2. Right frontal sinus
3. Brain stem and cerebellum
4. Pituitary gland
5. Right trigeminal nerve
6. Nose
7. Neck
8. Right eye
9. Right ear
11. trapezius muscle (neck, shoulder)
12. thyroid gland
13. parathyroid gland
36. reproductive gland (ovary or testis)

14. lung, bronchus
15. stomach
16. duodenum
17. pancreas
20. celiac plexus
21. adrenal gland
22. kidney
23. ureter
24. urinary bladder
25. small intestine
29. transverse colon
30. descending colon
31. rectum
32. anus
33. heart
34. spleen

3. Lateral side of foot: Diagram of reflecting area

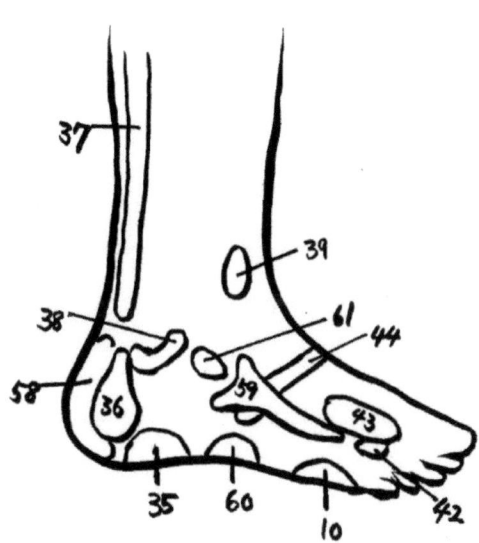

Fig.3 Reflecting areas on Lateral side of foot

10. shoulder
35. knee
36. reproductive gland
37. lower abdomen
38. hip joint
39.lymph nodes
(upper body)

42. balance organ
(labyrinth)
43. chest
44. diaphragm
58. sciatic nerve
59. scapula
60. elbow joint
61. ribs

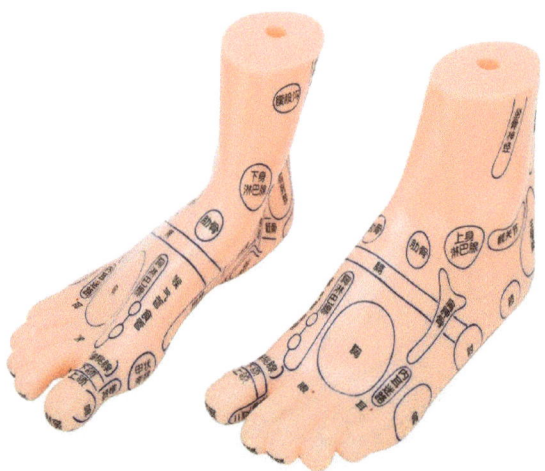

4. Medial side of foot: Diagram of reflecting area

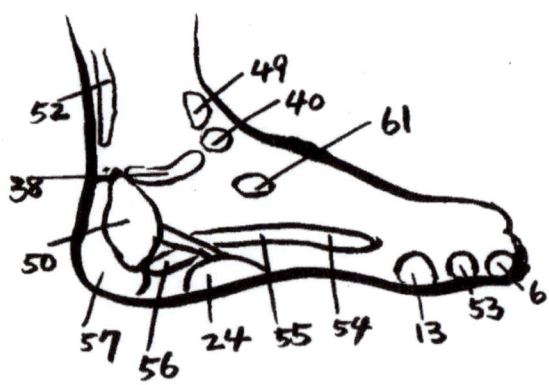

Fig. 4 Reflecting areas on Medial side of foot

6. nose

13. parathyroid gland

24. urinary bladder

38. hip joint

40. lymph nodes
(abdomen)

49. inguinal groove

50. uterus, prostate
gland

51. penis, vagina,
urethra

52. anus rectum
(hemorrhoid)

53. cervical spine

54. thoracic spine

55. lumbar spine

56. sacrum

57. coccyx

61. ribs

5. Dorsal side of foot: Diagram of reflecting areas

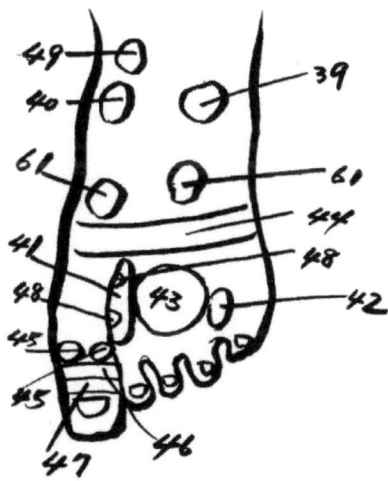

Fig. 5 Reflecting areas on Dorsal side of foot

39. lymph nodes (upper body)
40. lymph nodes (abdomen)
41. lymph nodes (chest)
42. balance organ (labyrinth)
43. chest
44. diaphragm
45. tonsils
46. lower jaw
47. palate
48. larynx, trachea, vocal cords
49. inguinal groove
61. ribs

Chapter 2. Foot Meridian Acupuncture

Foot acupuncture is traditional acupuncture, it is adopted according to the meridian theories and based on the close relationships between foot and meridians, internal organs, and Qi and blood to treat diseases by stimulating the circulation of Qi, adjusting vital energy, and expelling pathogens.

1. Method of localizing foot acupuncture points

1. Proportional bone measurement

(1) The distance between the heel border and the root of 3rd toe is divided into 10cun.

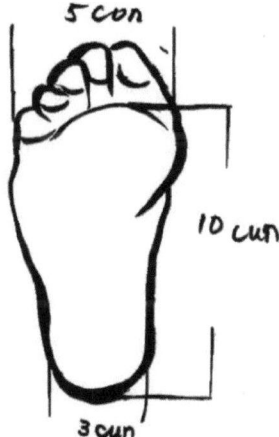

Fig. 1 Proportional bone measurement for sole

(2) The distance from tip of medial of lateral malleolus to medial or lateral border of foot is divided into 3 cun.

(3) The distance between medial border of first metatarsophalangeal joint and lateral border of 5th metatarsophalangeal joint on both dorsal and plantar side is divided into 5 cun.

(4) The widest part of the heel is divided into 3 cun.

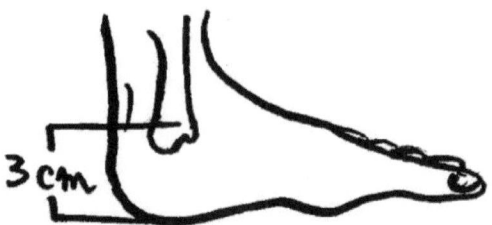

Fig. 2 Proportional bone measurement for side of foot

2. Surface anatomical landmarks

The acupuncture points are located according to surface anatomical landmarks which are the creases of toes, tips of toes, metatarsophalangeal joints, capitula of metatarsal bones, terminals of creases between toes, tips of medial and lateral malleoli, and tuberosity of navicular bone.

I. Foot Meridian

The foot has three Yin meridians and three Yang meridians.
Yin meridians: Spleen, Kidney, Liver.
Yang meridians: Stomach, Bladder, Gallbladder.

II. Foot Meridian Acupuncture points

1. The Spleen Channel of Foot-Taiyin
足太阴脾经经穴

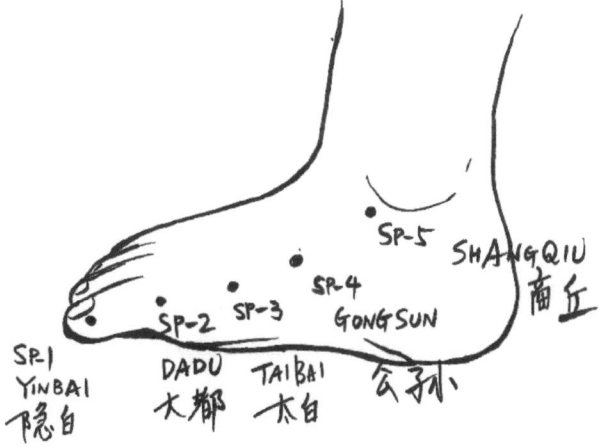

SP-1 (Yinbai 隱白)

- **Jing-Well point.**

Location

On the medial side of the big toe, 0.1 cun beside the corner of the nail.

Indications

Abdominal distension, apoplexy, convulsion, mental disorders, metrorrhagia, uterine bleeding, bloody stools.

SP-2 (Dadu 大都)

Location

On the medial side of the big toe, in the depression distal and inferior to the first metatarso-phalangeal joint.

Indications

Abdominal pain and distension, vomiting, diarrhea, febrile disease, constipation, dysphoria.

SP-3 (Taibai 太白)

- **Yuan -Source point of the Spleen channel.**

Location

On the medial side of the foot, in the depression proximal and inferior to the first metatarso-phalangeal joint.

Indications

Abdominal distension, stomachache, vomiting, diarrhea, constipation, edema, pain of joints, beriberi, heaviness of the body.

SP-4 (Gongsun 公孙)

- **Luo-Connecting point of the Spleen** channel.

Location

On the medial side of the foot, in the depression distal and inferior to the base of the first metatarsal bone.

Indications

Abdominal distension, diarrhea, edema, vomiting, dysentery, stomachache, insomnia, dysphoria, borborygmus.

SP-5 (Shangqiu 商丘)

Location

On the medial side of the foot, in the depression distal and inferior to the medial malleolus, the midpoint.

Indications

Abdominal distension, constipation, diarrhea, borborygmus, stiffness and pain of the tongue, hemorrhoid, pain in the foot and ankle.

2. The Liver Channel of Foot-Jueyin
足厥阴肝经经穴

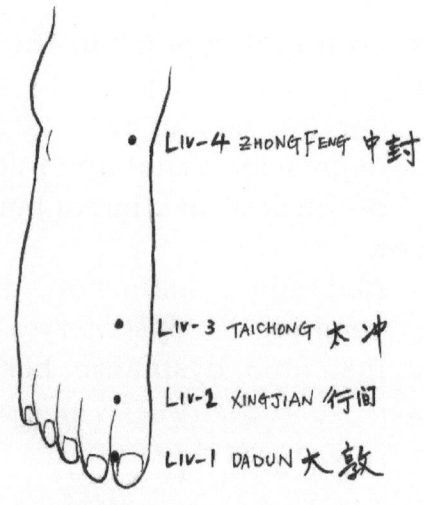

LIV-1 (Dadun 大敦)
- **Jing-Well point.**

Location

> On the lateral side of dorsum of the great toe, 0.1 cun beside the corner of the nail.

Indications

> Apoplexy, epilepsy, hernia, coma, irregular menstruation, metrorrhagia, metrostaxis, contraction of genitalia.

LIV-2 (Xingjian 行间)

Location

> On the lateral side of dorsum of the foot, between the first and second toes, 0.5 cun proximal of the margin of the web.

Indications

> Abdominal distension, headache, vertigo, redness and swelling pain of eyes, glaucoma, hernia, jaundice, irregular menstruation, metrorrhagia, metrostaxis, epilepsy, insomnia, pain and swelling in the dorsum of foot, numbness of toes.

LIV-3 (Taichong 太冲)

- **Yuan-Source of the Liver channel.**

Location

On the dorsum of the foot, in the depression distal to the junction, between the first and second metatarsal bones.

Indications

Headache, vertigo, dizziness, pain and swelling of the eyes, glaucoma, nearsightedness, facial paralysis, hernia, vomiting, pain in the hypochondriac region, epilepsy, apoplexy, flaccidity of lower limbs, severe lumbago, infantile convulsion.

LIV-4 (Zhongfeng 中封)

Location

On the ankle, anterior to the medial malleolus, in the depression on the medial side of the tendon of the m. tibialis anterior.

Indications

Hernia, retention of urine, metrorrhagia, metrostaxis, irregular menstruation, jaundice.

3. The Kidney Channel of Foot-Shaoyin
足少阴肾经经穴

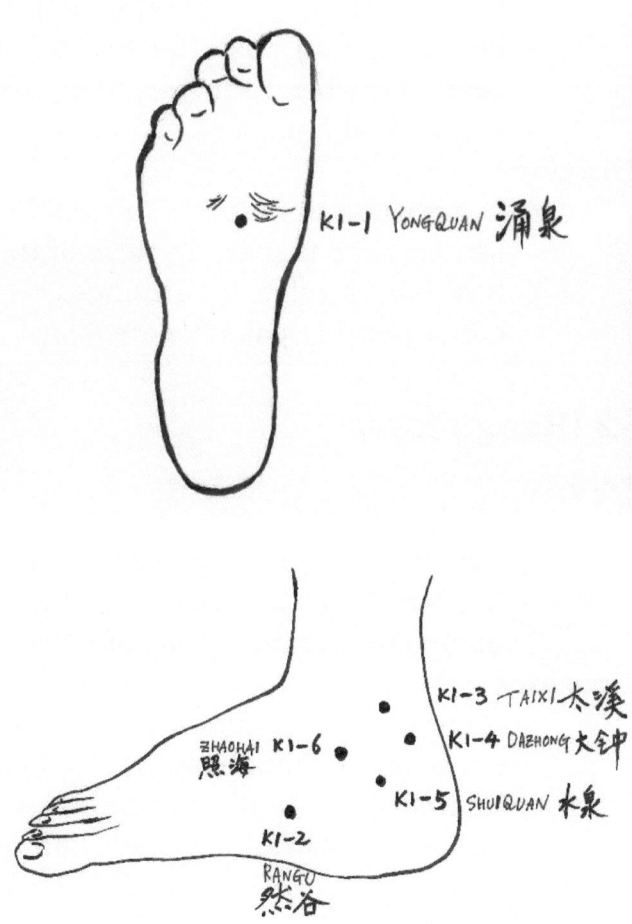

KI-1 (Yongquan 涌泉)

- **Jing-Well point.**

Location

> On the sole, at the junction of the anterior one-third and posterior two thirds of the sole, between the second and third metatarsal bones.

Indications

> Depression, mania, headache, wind stroke, sore throat, dryness of the tongue, feverish soles, dizziness, vertigo, constipation, loss of voice.

KI-2 (Rangu 然谷)

Location

> Anterior and inferior to the medial malleolus, in the depression on the lower border of the tuberosity of the navicular bone. constipation, loss of voice.

Indications

> Headache, dizziness, sore throat, irregular menstruation, leukorrhea, unsmooth urination, seminal emission, pain of the dorsum of foot, hemoptysis.

KI-3 (Taixi 太溪)

- **Yuan-Source of the Kidney channel.**

Location

On the medial malleolus, in the depression between the prominence of the medial malleolus and the Achilles tendon.

Indications

Tinnitus, deafness, headache, vertigo, sore throat, toothache, irregular menstruation, cough, asthma, seminal emission, impotence, pain in the heel, insomnia.

KI-4 (Dazhong 大钟)

- **Luo-Connecting point of the Kidney channel.**

Location

0.5 cun below posterior to KI-3 (Taixi 太溪), on the anterior border of the medial side of the tendon calcaneus.

Indications

Asthma, cough, dementia, dysuria, enuresis, frequent urination, pain in the heel, pain of the lower back.

KI-5 (Shuiquan 水泉)

- **Xi-Cleft point of the Kidney channel.**

Location

1 cun directly below KI-3 (Taixi 太溪), in the depression of the medial side of the tuberosity of the calcaneum.

Indications

Irregular menstruation, dysmenorrhea, blurred vision, unsmooth urination.

KI-6 (Zhaohai 照海)

Location

1 cun below the prominence of the medial malleolus.

Indications

Depression, mania, irregular menstruation, dysmenorrhea, insomnia, sore throat, constipation, pain and swelling in the malleolus joint.

4. The Stomach Channel of Foot-Yangming 足阴明胃经经穴

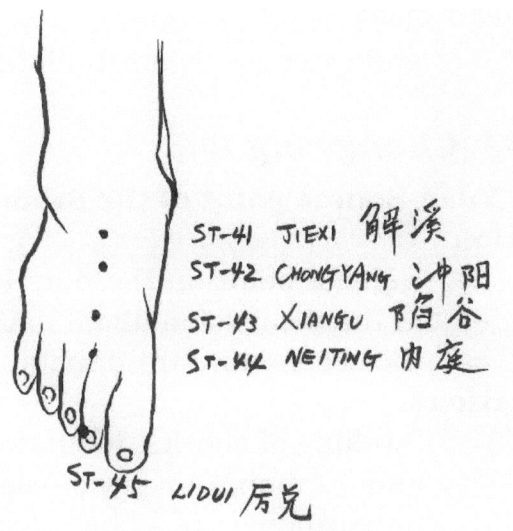

ST-41 JIEXI 解溪
ST-42 CHONGYANG 冲阳
ST-43 XIANGU 陷谷
ST-44 NEITING 内庭
ST-45 LIDUI 厉兑

ST-41 (Jiexi 解溪)

Location

Midpoint of the dorsum of the foot at the transverse malleolus, in a depression between the tendons of extensor hallucis longus and extensor digitorum longus.

Indications

Headache, vertigo, constipation, abdominal distension, epilepsy, swelling and pain of ankle joint, paralysis of the lower extremities, muscular atrophy, depressive and manic psychosis. longus and extensor digitorum longus.

ST-42 (Chongyang 冲阳)

- **Yuan-Source point of the Stomach channel.**

Location

Highest point on the dorsum of the foot, in the depression distal to the junction of the second and third metatarsal bones.

Indications

Swelling of cheeks, toothache, depressive and manic psychosis, epilepsy, impairment of the foot, epilepsy, muscular atrophy, epilepsy, flaccidity of foot.

ST-43 (Xiangu 陷谷)

Location

On the dorsum of the foot, between the second and third metatarsal bones, 1 cun proximal to ST-44 (Neiting 内庭).

Indications

Abdominal pain, swelling of cheeks, pain of the eyes, febrile disease, swelling and pain of the dorsum of foot.

ST-44 (Neiting 内庭)

Location

On the dorsum of the foot, between the second and third toes, at the end of the vertical skin crease of the web.

Indications

Toothache, pain in the face, sore throat, stomachache, epistaxis, abdominal distension, constipation, dysentery, diarrhea, swelling and pain of dorsum of foot, febrile disease. Vertical skin crease of the web.

ST-45 (Lidui 厉兑)

- **Jing-Well point.**

Location

On the lateral side of the 2nd toe, 0.1 cun beside the corner of the nail.

Indications

Toothache, facial swelling, sore throat, epistaxis, Mania, febrile disease.

5. The Bladder Channel of Foot-Taiyang

足太阴膀胱经经穴

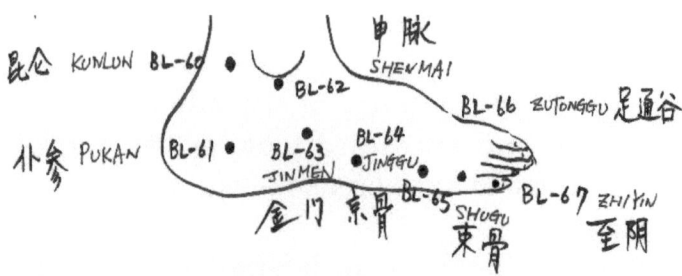

BL-60 (Kunlun 昆仑)

Location

Behind the ankle joint, in the depression between the prominence of the lateral malleolus.

Indications

Headache, dizziness, blurring vision, pain and swelling of the heel, low back pain, epilepsy, epistaxis.

BL-61 (Pucan 仆参)

Location

On the lateral side of the foot, directly below BL-60 (Kunlun 昆仑).

Indications

Pain in the heel, epilepsy, muscular atrophy, weakness of the lower extremities.

BL-62 (Shenmai 申脉)

Location

On the lateral side of the foot, directly below the lateral malleolus.

Indications

Epilepsy, mania, headache, dizziness, insomnia, aching of the leg.

BL-63 (Jinmen 金门)

- **Xi-Cleft point of the Bladder channel.**

Location

On the lateral side of the foot, in the depression below the cuboid bone which lies between the heel bone and the tuberosity of the 5th metatarsal bone.

Indications

Headache, epilepsy, mania, pain in the external malleolus, flaccidity and motor impairment of lower limbs.

BL-64 (Jinggu 京骨)

- **Yuan-Source point of the Bladder** channel.

Location

On the lateral side of the foot, in the depression below the tuberosity of the 5th metatarsal bone.

Indications

Headache, stiffness of neck, pain in the lower back and thigh, epilepsy, cataract.

BL-65 (Shugu 束骨)

Location

On the lateral side of the foot, posterior to the fifth metatarsal bone.

Indications

Headache, stiffness of neck, dizziness, manic depression, pain in the lower extremities, blurred vision.

BL-66 (Zutonggu 足通谷)

Location

On the lateral side of the foot, anterior to the fifth metatarso-phalangeal bone.

Indications

Headache, stiffness of neck, dizziness, manic, depression, epistaxis.

BL-67 (Zhiyin 至阴)

- **Jing-Well point.**

Location

> On the lateral side of the small toe, about 0.1 cun from the corner of the nail.

Indications

> Headache, epistasis, pain of eyes, malposition of fetus, nasal obstruction, dystocia, feverish sensation in the sole.

6. The Gallbladder Channel of Foot-Shaoyang 足少阴胆经经穴

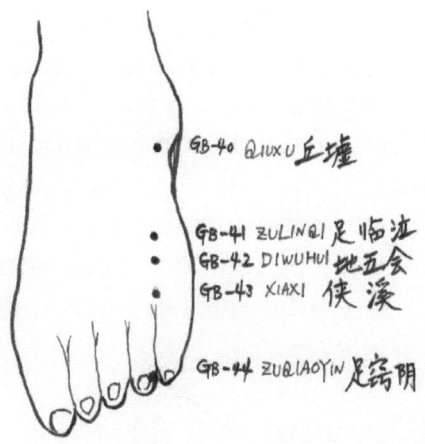

GB-40 (Qiuxu 丘墟)

- **Yuan-Source point of the Gall Bladder channel.**

Location

At the ankle joint, anterior and inferior to the lateral malleolus.

Indications

Pain in the hypochondriac region, vomiting acid regurgitation, muscular atrophy of the lower limbs, malaria, swelling and pain of the external malleolus.

GB-41 (Zulinqi 足临泣)

Location

On the lateral side of the dorsum of the foot, 4th and 5th metatarsal bones, in a depression lateral to the tendon of the extensor digitiform longus of the fifth toe.

Indications

Hypochondriac pain, numbness of toes, pain of foot dorsum, numbness of toes, irregular menstruation, pain and swelling of eyes.

GB-42 (Diwuhui 地五会)

Location

Between the 4th and 5th metatarsal bones, on the medial side of the tendon of extensor digitorum longus.

Indications

Pain of the canthus, tinnitus, swelling and pain of foot dorsum, distending pain of the breast.

GB-43 (Xiaxi 侠溪)

Location

Between the fourth and fifth toes, 0.5 cun proximal to the margin of the web.

Indications

Headache, vertigo, tinnitus, deafness, swelling and pain of the eyes, pain in the hypochondria, distending pain of the breast, febrile diseases.

GB-44 (Zuqiaoyin 足窍阴)

- **Jing-Well point.**

Location

On the lateral side of the fourth toe, 0.1 cun from the corner of the nail.

Indications

Headache, redness, swelling and pain of eyes, migraine, deafness, tinnitus, febrile diseases, insomnia, hypochondriac pain apoplexy, sore throat.

7. Extra Foot Acupuncture points 常用经外奇穴定位

EX-LE7 (Neihuaijian 内踝尖)

Location

On the medial side of the foot, at the prominence of the medial malleolus.

Indications

Pain and paralysis of the lower extremities, muscular atrophy.

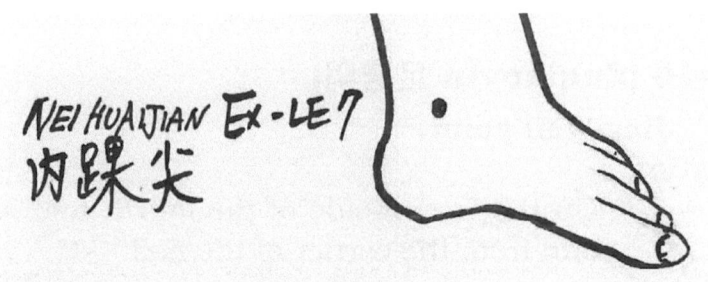

EX-LE8 (Waihuaijian 外踝尖)

Location

On the lateral side of the foot, at the prominence of the lateral malleolus.

Indications

Pain and paralysis of the lower extremities, muscular atrophy.

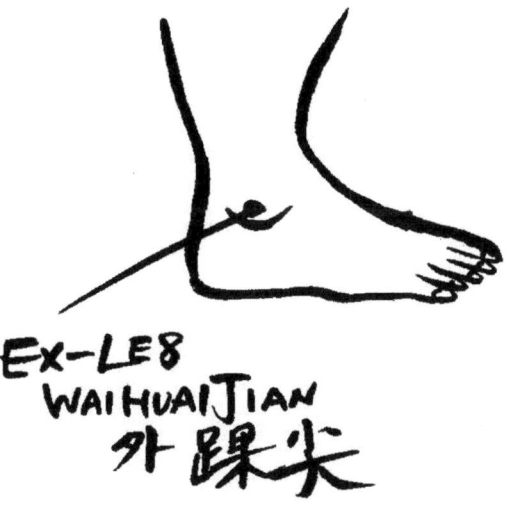

EX-LE8
WAIHUAIJIAN
外踝尖

EX-LE9 (Bafeng 八风)

Location

On the dorsum of the foot, at the margin of the webs between each two toes, four points on each foot, eight points in all.

Indications

Toe pain, redness and swelling of the dorsum of the foot, numbness of the lower limb.

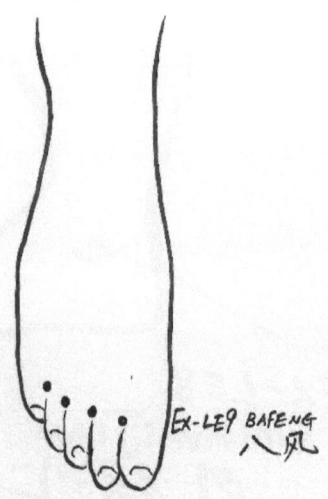

EX-LE9 BAFENG 八风

EX-LE10 (Duyin 独阴)

Location

On the plantar side of the second toe, at the midpoint of the transverse crease.
Indications
Pain, redness and swelling of the foot, muscular atrophy, pain, and numbness of the lower limb.

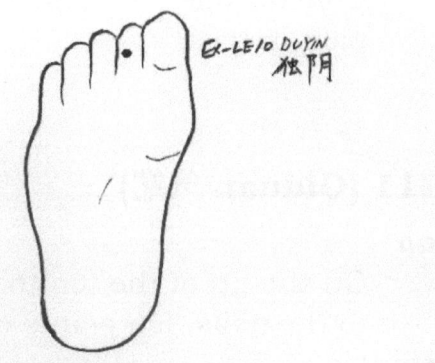

EX (Lineiting 里内庭)

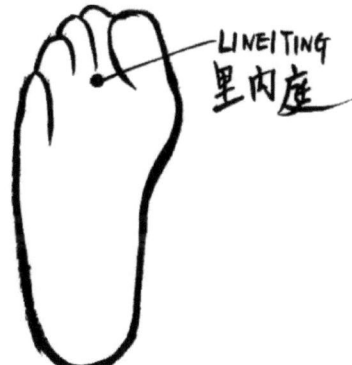

Location

On the plantar side of foot, in the depression between the second and third toe and on the opposite side of ST-44 (Neiting 内庭).

Indications

Convulsions in children, epilepsy, and pain in toes.

EX-LE11 (Qiduan 气端)

Location

On the tip of the ten toes, 0.1 cun distal to the nails, ten points in all.

Indications

Pain, redness and swelling of the foot, muscular atrophy, numbness of the lower limb.

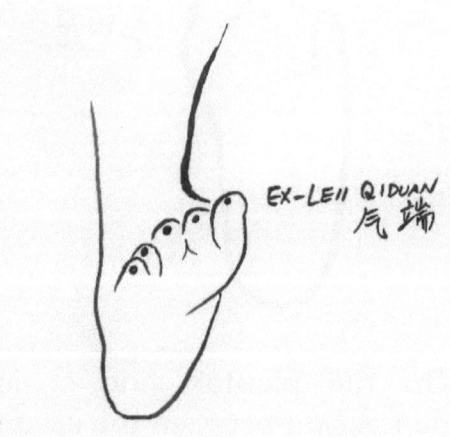

8. Other Extra Foot Acupuncture points
(1)

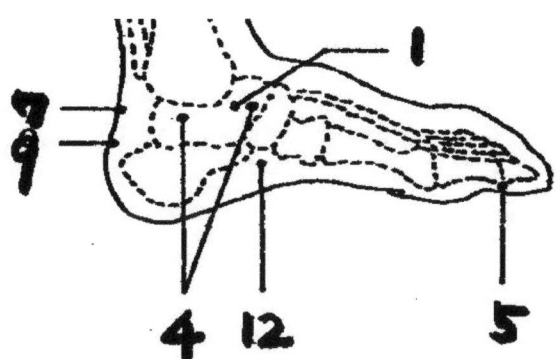

1.EX (Neihuai 内踝 Qianxia)
4. EX (Yingchi)
5. EX (Yinyang 阴阳)

7. EX (Quanshengzu)
9. EX (Shuwei)
12. EX (Ranhou)

1. EX-F1 (Neihuai Qianxia)
Location

One finger width anterior to the midpoint of lower border of medial malleolus.

Indications

Regurgitations of food.

4. EX-F4 (Yingchi)
Location

In the depressions anterior and posterior to the lower border of medial malleolus.

Indications

Profuse menstrual discharge and discharge of red and white leukorrhea.

5. EX-F5 (Yinyang 阴阳)
Location

At the medial end of the interphalangeal crease of big toe.

Indications

Syncope, diarrhea, discharge of red and white leukorrhea.

7. EX-F7 (Quanshengzu)
Location

On the posterior midline of Achilles tendon and at the midpoint of the crease above heel bone.

Indications

Spasm of esophagus, difficult labor, lumbago.

9. EX-F9 (Shuwei)
Location

At the midpoint of upper border of heel bone.

Indications

Tubercles of cervical lymph nodes.

12. EX-F12 (Ranhou)
Location

1.3 cm posterior to KI-2 (Rangu).

Indications

Indigestion.

(2)

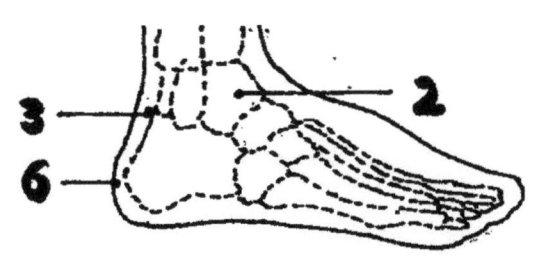

2. EX (Waihuaijian 外踝尖 Jiaomai)

3. EX (Xiakunlun 下昆仑)
6. EX (Nüxi)

2. EX-F2 (Waihuaijian 外踝尖 qian Jiaomai)
Location

On the dorsal side of ankle joint and at the junction of medial three fourths and lateral one fourth of a connecting line between the tips of medial and lateral malleolus.

Indications

Toothache.

3. EX-3 (Xiakunlun 下昆仑)

Location

On the anterior border of Achilles tendon and 3.3 cm below the tip of lateral malleolus.

Indications

Lumbago, migraine, hemiplegia, painful walking, Bi syndrome due to cold.

6. EX-F6 (Nüxi)
Location

At the midpoint of heel bone.

Indications

Mental diseases, vomiting, diarrhea, muscular spasms, convulsions.

(3)

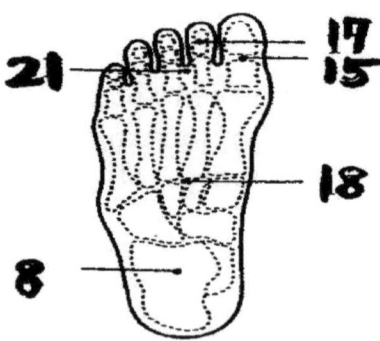

8. EX (Shimian 失眠)　　　　17. EX (duyin 独阴)
15. EX (Muzhi Lihengwen)　　18. EX (Zuxin)

21. EX (Lineiting 里内庭)

8. EX-F8 (Shimian 失眠)
Location

On the sole and at the crossing point of the midline of sole and the connecting line of medial and lateral malleolus.

Indications

Insomnia, pain of the sole

15. EX-F15 (Muzhi Lihengwen)
Location

On the platar side of big toe and at the midpoint of crease of interphalangeal joint.

Indications

Hernia.

17. EX-17 (Duyin 独阴)
Location

On the plantar side of foot and at the midpoint of the crease of 2nd metatarsophalangeal joint.

Indications

Hernia, irregular menstruation, pregnancy vomiting.

18. EX-18 (Zuxin)
Location

At the midpoint of a connecting line between the tip of 2nd toe and the posterior border of heel.

Indications

Headache, epilepsy, vertigo, pain of the sole.

21. EX-F21 (Lineiting 里内庭)
Location

On the plantar side of foot, between the 2nd and 3rd toes, and on the opposite side of ST-44 (Neiting 内庭).

Indications

Epilepsy, pain in toes, convulsions in children.

(4)

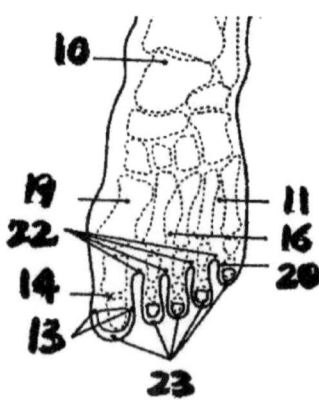

10. EX (Quchi 曲池)
11. EX (Tongli 通里)
14. EX (Dazhi Jumao)
16. EX (Erzhishang)
19. EX (Neitaichong 内太冲)
20. EX (Neizhiyin 内至阴)

13. EX (Jiagen)

22. EX (Bafeng 八风)
23. EX (Qiduan 气端)

10. EX (LI-11) (Quchi 曲池)
Location

On the medial side of foot arch, below and anterior to medial malleolus and in a depression between the tendons of anterior tibial muscle and long extensor muscle of big toe.

Indications

Hernia, pain in lower abdomen.

11. EX (HT-5) (Tongli 通里)
Location

On the dorsum of foot and 1.6 cm anterior to the posterior end of the interosseous space between 4th and 5th metatarsal bones.

Indications

Profuse menstrual discharge.

13. EX-11 (Jiagen)

Location

On the dorsal side of big toe and beside the medial and lateral corners of nail.

Indications

Hernia.

14. EX-14 (Dazhi Jumao)

Location

On the dorsal side of big toe and in the hair on the interphalangeal joint of this toe.

Indications

Hernia, vertigo, headache, apoplexy with coma.

16. EX-16 (Erzhishang)

Location

At the midpoint between ST-44 (Neiting 内庭) and ST-43 (Xiangu 陷谷).

Indications

Edema.

19. EX-F19 (Neitaichong 内太冲)

Location

On the dorsal side of foot, in a depression on the tibial side of tendon of long extensor muscle of big toe and on the opposite side of Liv-3 (Taichong 太冲).

Indications

Hernia.

20. EX-20 (Neizhiyin 内至阴)

Location

0.3 cm from the medial corner of nail of little toe, and opposite BL-67 (Zhiyin 至阴).

Indications

Hysteria, convulsions in children.

22. EX-LE10 (Bafeng 八风)

Location

On the dorsum of foot, between all toes and on the dorsoplantar boundary of the web folds.

Indications

Headache, toothache, irregular menstruation.

23. EX-LE12 (Qiduan 气端)

Location

On the tips of all ten toes.

Indications

Beriberi, paralysis of toes, sudden treatment.

Chapter 3. Foot Acupuncture Therapy

1. Foot Acupuncture

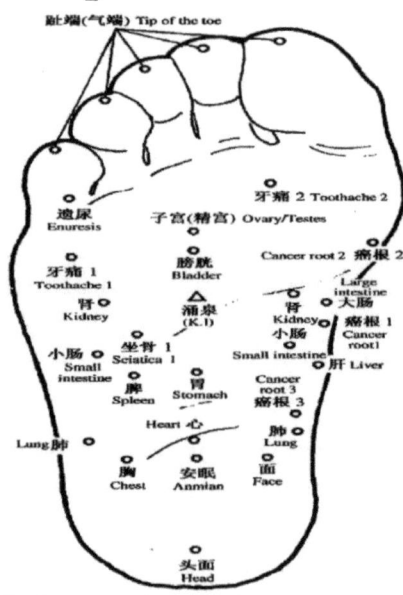

趾端(气端) Tip of the toe

遗尿 Enuresis

子宫(精宫) Ovary/Testes

牙痛 2 Toothache 2

牙痛 1 Toothache 1

膀胱 Bladder

Cancer root 2 癌根 2

肾 Kidney

涌泉 (K.1)

肾 Kidney
小肠 Small intestine

Large intestine 大肠

癌根 1 Cancer root1

小肠 Small intestine

坐骨 1 Sciatica 1

Small intestine

肝 Liver

脾 Spleen

胃 Stomach

Cancer root 3 癌根 3

Heart 心

Lung 肺

肺 Lung

胸 Chest

安眠 Anmian

面 Face

头面 Head

Foot acupuncture point

• Effectiveness

(1) Balance adjustment of Yin and Yang.

(2) Release of stasis of meridians by applying acupuncture and moxibustion.

(3) Improve body resistance and discharge pathogens.

(1). Acupuncture on the Sole

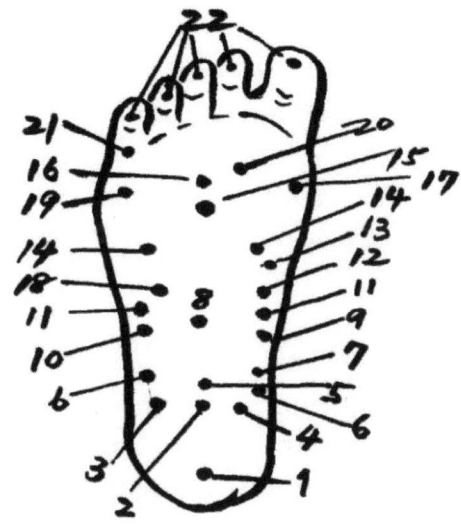

On the Sole

1. Head and face
2. Anmian
3. Chest
4. Face
5. Heart
6. Lung
7. Aigen 3
8. Stomach
9. Liver
10. Spleen
11. Small Intestine

12. Aigen 1
13. Colon
14. Kidney
15. Bladder
16. Uterus
17. Aigen 2
18. Ischium 1
19. Toothache 1
20. Toothache 2
21. Bed-wetting
22. Zhiduan

1. Head and face
Location

On the midline and 1 cun from the posterior heel border.

Indications

Common cold, headache, maxillary sinusitis, and rhinitis.

2. Anmian
Location

On the midline, 3 cun from the posterior heel border and at the midpoint on the connecting line of medial and lateral malleoli.

Indications

Insomnia, psychosis, hysteria, neurasthenia, hypotension.

3. Chest
Location

1 cun lateral to the midline of foot, 3 cun from the posterior heel border and 1 cun lateral to Anmian.

4. Face
Location

1 cun medial to Anmian.

Indications

Trigeminal neuralgia, facial palsy, facial itching.

5. Heart

Location

On the midline and 3.5 cun from the posterior border of heel.

Indications

Hypertension, heart palpitations, heart pain sore throat, stiff tongue, tongue pain, insomnia.

6. Lung

Location

1.5 cun on either side of heart.

Indications

Cough, asthma, chest pain.

7. Aigen 3

Location

1.5 cun medial to the midline of sole, 4cun from posterior heel border and 0.5 cun medial to lung.

Indications

Relief of pain, spasms, and other symptoms of cancers of nasopharynx, neck, lungs, upper and middle segment of esophagus.

8. Stomach
Location

On the midline of sole, 5 cun from the posterior heel border.

Indications

Vomiting, indigestion, insomnia.

9. Liver
Location

2 cun medial to stomach.

Indications

Hepatitis, cholecystitis, intercostal neuralgia, eye diseases.

10. Spleen
Location

1 cun lateral to stomach.

Indications

Indigestion, diarrhea, retention of urine, blood diseases, Insomnia.

11. Small intestine

Location

> 1.5 cun medial and lateral to the midline, 5.5 cun from posterior heel border.
> Indications
> Abdominal pain, diarrhea, intestinal gurgling, dysentery.

12. Aigen 1
Location

> 2 cun medial to the midline of sole, 6 cun from posterior heel border.

Indications

> Relief of pain, symptoms cancers of lower end of esophagus, stomach, cardia.

13. Colon
Location

> 2 cun medial to the midline of sole and 6.5 cun from posterior heel border.

Indications

> Abdominal pain, vomiting, diarrhea, dysentery.

14. Kidney
Location

> 1.5 cun medial and lateral to KI-1 (Yongquan 涌泉).

Indications

Headache, vertigo, psychosis, retention of urine, incontinence of urine, lumbago.

15. Bladder
Location

On the midline of sole and 2 cun posterior to the root of 3rd toe.

Indications

Retention of urine, bed-wetting, incontinence of urine.

16. Uterus
Location

On the midline of sole and 1.5 cun posterior to the root of 3rd toe.

Indications

Irregular menstruation, dysmenorrhea, leukorrhagia, retention of urine, orchitis.

17. Aigen 2
Location

2.5 cun medial to urinary bladder.

Indications

Relief of pain, other symptoms of cancers in organs below umbilicus, metastatic tumors in lymph nodes.

18. Ischium
Location
>4 cun posterior to the root of 4th toe.

Indications
>Neuralgia sciatica, lumbago, urticaria, shoulder pain.

19. Toothache 1
Location
>1 cun posterior to the root of little toe.

Indications
>Toothache.

20. Toothache 2
Location
>1 cun posterior to the junction of the big and 2nd toes.

Indications
>Toothache.

21. Bed-wetting
Location
>At the midpoint of the crease of first interphalangeal joint of little toe.

Indications
>Bed-wetting and frequent urination.

22. Tip of toes (Zhiduan 指端)

Location

At the tips of toes.

Indications

Apoplexy with coma, numbness of toes, gangrene of toes, and beriberi.

(2) Acupuncture on dorsum of foot

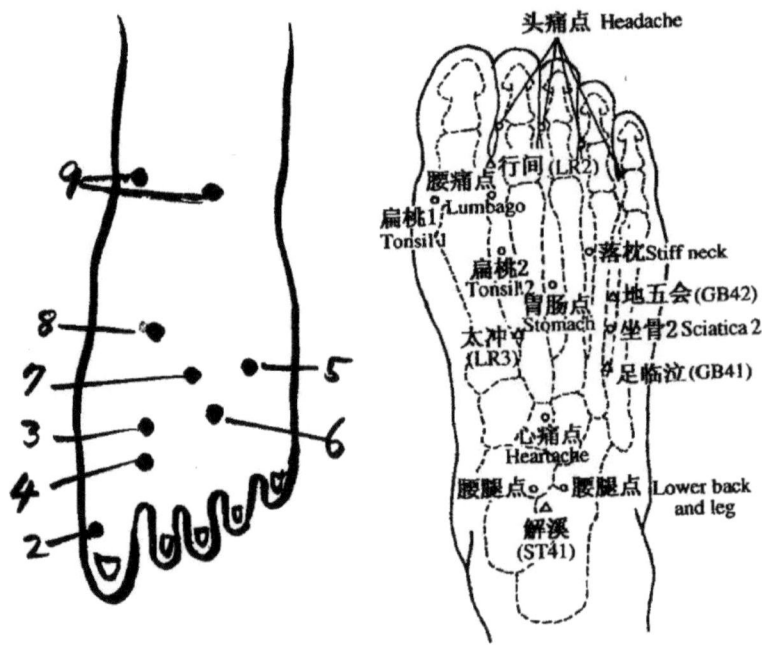

Points on the dorsum of Foot

2. Tonsil 1
3. Tonsil 2
4. Lumbago
5. Ischium 2
6. Stiff neck

7. Stomach and intestine
8. Heart pain
9. Waist and leg pain

2. Tonsil 1
Location

On the big toe, at the metatarsophalangeal joint and medial to the tendon of long extensor muscle of the big toe.

Indications

Acute tonsillitis, epidemic parotitis, eczema, and urticaria.

3. Tonsil 2
Location

At the midpoint between Liv-3 (Taichong 太冲) and Liv-2 (Xingjian 行间).

Indications

Acute tonsillitis and epidemic parotitis.

4. Lumbago
Location

In a depression lateral to the capitulum of first metatarsal bone.

Indications

Acute waist sprain and lumbago.

5. Ischium 2

Location

On the dorsum of foot, at the midpoint, between GB41 (Zulinqi 足临泣) and GB-42 (Diwuhui 地五会).

Indications

Neuralgia sciatica.

6. Stiff neck

Location

On the dorsum of foot, 2 cun behind the junction of 3rd and 4th toes.

Indications

Stiff neck.

7. Stomach and intestine

Location

On the dorsum of foot, 3 cun behind the junction of 2nd and 3rd toes.

Indications

Gastroenteritis, gastric duodenal peptic ulcer.

8. Heart pain

Location

2.5 cun below ST-41 (Jiexi 解溪).

Indications

Heart pain, heart palpitations, asthma, common cold.

9. Waist and leg pain

Location

0.5 cun below ST-41 (Jiexi 解溪) in bilateral depressions.

Indications

Lumbago, pain and spasm of lower limb.

(3) Acupuncture on medial side of foot

1. Vertigo
2. Dysmenorrhea 1
3. Dysmenorrhea 2
4. Epilepsy

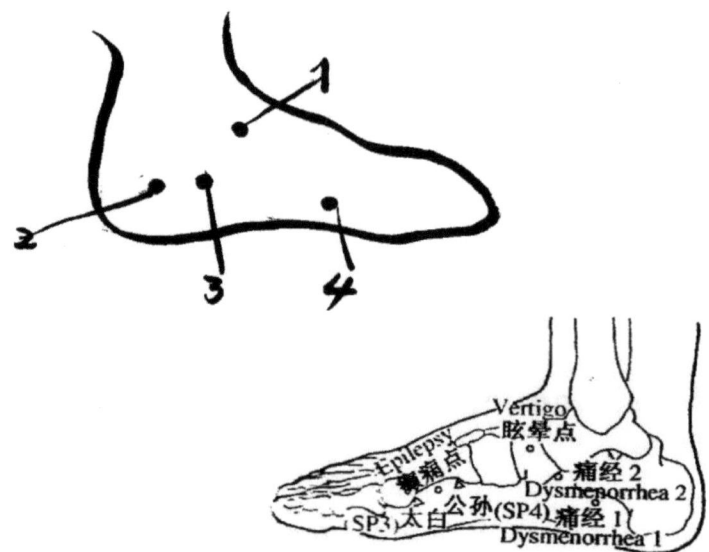

Points on the medial side of the foot

1. Vertigo
Location

On the medial side of foot, in a depression above tuberosity of navicular bone.

Indications

Vertigo, headache, hypertension, parotitis, tonsilitis.

2. Dysmenorrhea 1
Location

2 cun directly below the tip of medial malleolus.

Indications

Irregular menstruation, dysmenorrhea, uterine bleeding.

3. Dysmenorrhea 2

Location

On the medial side of foot, in a depression below and behind the tuberosity of navicular bone.

Indications

Dysmenorrhea, uterine bleeding.

4. Epilepsy

Location

At the midpoint between SP-3 (Taibai 太白) and SP-4 (Gongsun 公孙).

Indications

Epilepsy, hysteria, neurasthenia.

(4) Acupuncture on Lateral side of foot

1. Buttocks

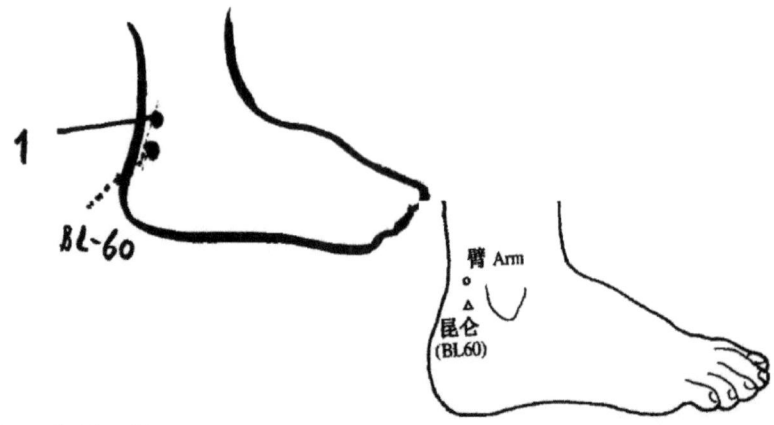

Lateral side of foot

1. buttocks
Location
1 cun above BL-60 (Kunlun 昆仑).
Indications
Sciatica, headache, abdominal pain.

Chapter 4. Other Foot Therapy Methods

1. Foot Massage

Tuina is TCM traditional massage. The foot has a compact structure of bones and muscles.

- **Effectiveness**

(1) Balances of Yin and Yang, adjustment of internal organs.

(2) Promotes blood circulation and relieves blood stasis.

(3) Relaxes the muscle and tranquilizes the mind.

(4) It is safe and effective without harm and pain.

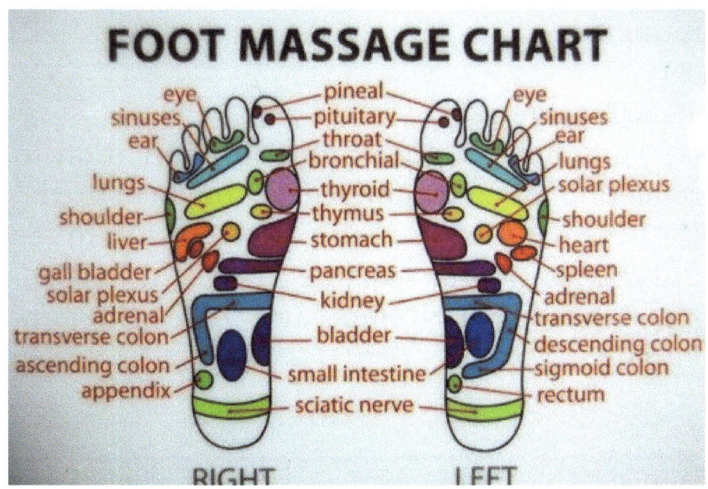

2. Foot Bath

This is an external TCM therapy, which is the streaming and washing method, the feet are placed in stream evaporated from a boiled herbal decoction for the treatment of disease. This affects Qi, blood, and the meridians from the body surface to the internal organs. This reinforces Qi and blood, Yin and Yang, and removes pathogens.

3. Application of Drugs on Foot

This combination of drugs made of Chinese herbs is applied over the reflecting areas and foot acupuncture.

- **Effectiveness**
(1) This may produce a direct stimulation to the reflecting areas by application on local area.
(2) They are absorbed through the skin to resolve inflammation and swelling.
(3) Expels cold, damp, and relieves pain and fatigue.

Chapter 5. Treatment of common diseases

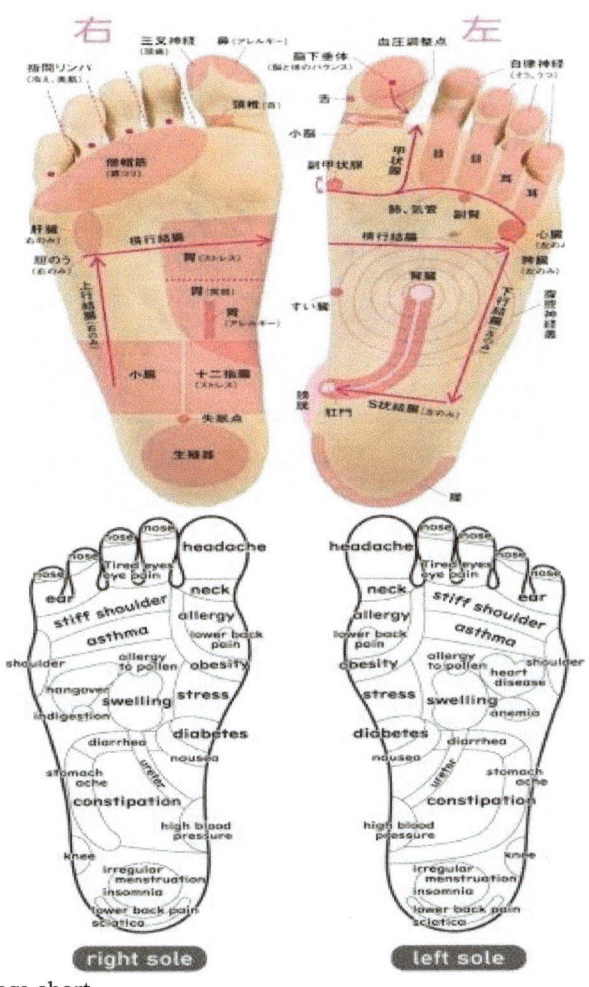

Foot massage chart

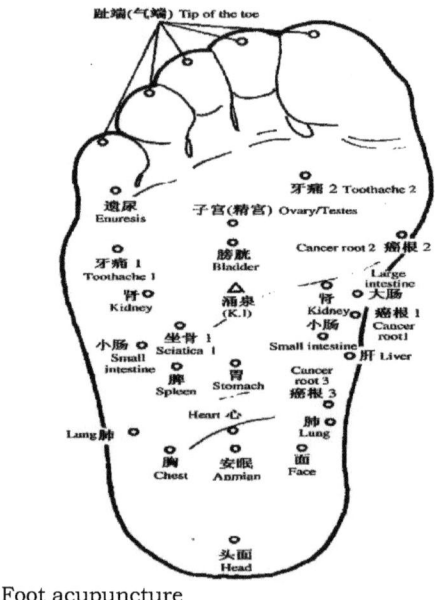

Foot acupuncture

I. Internal Medicine

I-1 Asthma 哮喘 Xiaochuan

It is characterized by paroxysmal attacks of gasping, difficulty breathing, and a whistling noise in the throat. It is caused by an accumulation of phlegm, constriction of the respiratory tract, and interference with pulmonary ventilation producing gasps and a whistling sound.

- **Treatment**
1. Foot meridian acupuncture:
GB-41 (Zulinqi 足临泣), BL-60 (Kunlun 昆仑),
BL66 (Zutonggu 足通谷), SP-1 (Yinbai 隐白), KI-1
(Yongquan 涌泉), KI-2 (Rangu 然谷)
2. Foot acupuncture: Chest, Aigen 3, heart pain,
Kidney
3. Foot massage: Larynx, Trachea, Vocal cord,
Lung and Bronchus, Lymph nodes, Parathyroid
gland, Kidney, Spleen, Adrenal gland

I-2 Bi syndrome 痹症 Bizheng

This is characterized by numbness, heaviness,
limited movement, swollen joints. This is caused by
the attack of wind, cold, heat and damp pathogens
blocking the meridians.

- **Treatment**
1. Foot meridian acupuncture:
ST-41 (Jiexi 解溪), BL-60 (Kunlun 昆仑), BL-61
(Pucanpucan 仆参), BL-62 (Shenmai 申脉), BL-63
(Jinmen 金门), SP-5 (Shangqiu 商丘), EX

(Xiakunlun 下昆仑) (under BL-60 Kunlun 昆仑),
EX-LE11 (Qiduan 气端)
2. Foot massage: Spleen, Stomach, Kidney, Lung,
Lymph nodes (upper body, abdomen chest),
Adrenal gland

I-3 Constipation 便秘 Bianmi

This is characterized by hard stools difficult to pass,
and prolonged intervals between bowel movements.

- **Treatment**
1. Foot meridian acupuncture:
ST-41 ((Jiexi 解溪), ST-44 (Neiting 内庭), SP-4
(Gongsun 公孙), SP-5 (Shangqiu 商丘), KI-2 (Rangu
然谷)
2. Foot massage: Rectum, Anus, Colon
(ascending, transverse, descending)

I-4 Cervical spondylosis 颈椎病 Jingchuibing

Pain in the around the neck, forearm, shoulder, movement of the head, numbness in the lower limbs, heavy sensation, dizziness, headache.

(1) Nerve root type
Neck pain, shoulder and occipital region stiffness and limitation of neck movement, radiating pain to shoulder and arm on one side.

(2) Sympathetic nerve type
Occipital region pain, dizziness, migraine, dilatation of one pupil.

- **Treatment**
1. Foot meridian acupuncture:
(1) For nerve root type
BL-60 (Kunlun 昆仑), BL-65 (Shugu 束骨), ST-45 (Lidui 厉兑), GB-40 (Qiuxu 丘墟)

(2) Sympathetic nerve type
BL-66 (Zutonggu 足通谷), BL-67 (Zhiyin 至阴), GB-41 (Zulinqi 足临泣), ST-41 (Jiexi 解溪), BL-64 (Jinggu 京骨)

2. Foot massage: Cervical Spine, Neck, Elbow joint, Trapezius muscle, Frontal sinus, Scapula, Shoulder

I-5 Car sickness 晕车 Yunche

This is characterized by dizziness, headache, nausea, vomiting.

- **Treatment**
1. Foot meridian acupuncture:
KI-1 (Yongquan 涌泉), ST-41 (Jiexi 解溪), KI-4 (Dazhong 大钟), SP-3 (Taibai 太白), SP-2 (Dadu 大都)
2. Foot massage: Head, Brain stem balance organ (labyrinth)

I-6 Common cold 普通感冒 Putongganmao

The Main manifestations are high fever without sweating, headache, fullness sensation in the chest, lassitude, nausea, anorexia, abdominal distention, loose stool, sticky whitish sputum, thick yellow tongue coating, soft rapid pulse.

- **Treatment**
1. Foot meridian acupuncture:
BL-60 (Kunlun 昆仑), ST-41 (Jiexi) 解溪), BL-66 (Zutonggu 足通谷), KI-6 (Zhaohai 照海), KI-2

(Rangu 然谷), EX (Dazhi Jumao), EX (Zuxin), EX-LE-9 (Bafeng 八风)

2. Foot acupuncture:
Head and face, Kidney, Heart pain
3. Foot massage:
Head, cerebellum, throat, tonsil, nose

I-7 Cough 咳嗽 Kesou

- **Differentiation**

1. Exopathogenic Factors
(1) Wind-Cold Type
It is characterized by itching sensation in the throat. It is accompanied by fever, chills, headache, nasal obstruction, soreness of joints. The tongue has thin white coating, and superficial pulse.

(2) Wind-Heat Type
Fever without chills, thirst, cough with thick sputum, dry mouth and sticky yellowish sputum, tongue with yellowish coating, rapid superficial pulse.

2. Endopathogenic Factors
(1) Yang Deficiency with Spleen
Cough with excessive sputum, fullness sensation in the chest and epigastric region, listlessness, white greasy tongue coating, deep and slow pulse.

(2) Yin Deficiency with Dryness of the Lung
Dry cough without sputum, dry throat, feverish palms and soles, fever, red tongue with thin coating, feeble rapid pulse.

- **Treatment**
  1. Foot meridian acupuncture:
  GB-44 (Zuqiaoyin 足窍阴), BL-66 (Zutonggu 足通谷), KI-1 (Yongquan 涌泉), KI-3 (Taixi 太溪), KI-4 (Dazhong 大钟), ST-45 (Lidui 厉兑), ST-44 (Neiting 内庭), ST-42 (Chongyang 冲阳), ST-43 (Xiangu 陷谷)
  2. Foot acupuncture: Lung, Spleen, Stomach, Liver
  3. Foot massage: Larynx, Trachea, Vocal cord, Lung and Bronchus, Lymph nodes (chest), Kidney, Spleen

I-8 Diarrhea 泄泻 Xiexie

1. Acute Diarrhea
(1) Cold-Damp Type
Loose stools with abdominal pain, borborygmus, cold with desire for warmth, absence of thirst, pale tongue with white coating, deep and slow pulse.

(2) Damp-Heat Type
Loose stools with abdominal pain, urgent bowel motion, feverish sensation in the anus, scanty urine, yellow greasy tongue coating, rapid slippery, soft pulse.

1. Chronic Diarrhea
(1) Spleen Yang Deficiency
Loose stools with undigested food, abdominal and epigastric distension, anorexia, lassitude, white sticky tongue coating, soft slow pulse.

(2) Kidney Yang Deficiency
Abdominal pain, borborygmus and diarrhea before dawn, cold extremities, white tongue coating, deep forceless pulse.

- **Treatment**

1. Foot meridian acupuncture:
ST-41 (Jiexi 解溪), ST-44 (Neiting 内庭), ST-45 (Lidui 厉兑), KI-2 (Rangu 然谷), SP-1 (Yinbai 隐白), SP-2 (Dadu 大都), SP-4 (Gongsun 公孙), SP-5 (Shangqiu 商丘), EX (Yinyang), EX (Ranhou)

2. Foot massage: Spleen, stomach, liver, kidney colon (ascending, transverse and descending colon)

I-9 Diabetes mellitus 糖尿病 Tangniaobing

This is a metabolic and endocrine condition with disturbance of carbohydrate metabolism due to functional reduction of pancreatic islets with increase of appetite and profuse discharge of urine, loss of body weight, and complications of hypertension, coronary heart disease, cerebral hemorrhage, cerebral thrombosis, cerebral embolism, gangrene of limbs.

- **Differentiation**

(1) Upper Diabetes

Thirst, dry mouth, profuse urination, polydipsia, red tip of the tongue, thin yellow tongue coating, full rapid pulse.

(2) Middle Diabetes

Polyphagia, easy hunger, restlessness, profuse sweating, emaciation, profuse drinking of water, polyuria, dry yellow tongue coating, slippery rapid pulse.

(3) Lower Diabetes

Profuse and frequent urination, turbid urine with sweet taste, thirst and polydipsia, dizziness, blurred vision, red cheeks, soreness and weakness of the knee, red tongue, thin and rapid pulse.

- **Treatment**

1. Foot meridian acupuncture:

KI-3 (Taixi 太溪), KI-2 (Rangu 然谷), Liv-2 (Xingjian 行间), KI-6 (Zhaohai 照海), Liv-4 (Zhongfeng 中封), SP-1 (Yinbai 隐白), SP-5 (Shangqiu 商丘)

2. Foot massage: Pancreas, Pituitary gland, Stomach, Kidney, Adrenal gland, Lung, Urinary bladder

I-10 Dysentery 痢疾 Liji

It is with symptoms of abdominal pain, tenesmus and diarrhea with blood and pus in stool.

- **Treatment**
1. Foot meridian acupuncture:
SP-4 (Gongsun 公孙), BL-65 (Shugu 束骨), ST-44 (Neiting 内庭), SP-3 (Taibai 太白), SP-5 (Shangqiu 商丘), KI-1 (Yongquan 涌泉)
2. Foot acupuncture:
Small intestine, Colon

I-11 Emission 排放 Paifang

Emission is a spontaneous discharge of semen without sexual activity.
This is characterized by dizziness, tinnitus, unstable sleep, lassitude, weakness of body.

- **Treatment**
1. Foot meridian acupuncture: SP-4 (Gongsun 公孙), BL-67 (Zhiyin 至阴), KI-2 (Rangu 然谷), KI-3 (Taixi 太溪), Liv-4 (Zhongfeng 中封), EX (Quchi)

2. Foot massage: Kidney, Liver, Spleen, Stomach, Heart

I-12 Epilepsy 癫痫 Dianxian

This is a neurological condition causing convulsions.

- **Differentiation**
1. During
Experiences headache, dizziness in the chest, followed by unconsciousness, pallor complexion, clenched jaws, the eyes staring upward, mouthful forms, sleep with big noise. In short time, patients become normal situation, white greasy tongue, thready slippery pulse.

2.After
Palpitation, Dizziness, listlessness, profuse sputum, lumbar soreness, knee weakness, pale white greasy tongue, thin, slippery pulse.

- **Treatment**
1. Foot meridian acupuncture:
ST-45 (Lidui 厉兑), Liv-2 (Xingjian 行间), BL-60 (Kunlun 昆仑), BL-61 (Pucan 仆参) BL-63 (Jinmen 金门), BL-65 (Shugu

束骨), ST-41 (Jiexi 解溪), EX (Zuxin), EX (Lineiting)

2. Foot acupuncture: Epilepsy, Heart, Spleen
3. Foot massage: Head, Brain stem and Cerebellum, Kidney, Heart, Spleen

I-13 Facial Spasm 面肌痉挛 Mianjijingluan

This is common in women and refers to spasm on one side of the face, and this is a condition of the facial muscles, automatic, irregular and paroxysmal spasms or twitching.

- **Differentiation**

It may be aggravated by fatigue, mental stress, and physical movement. Patients may be suffered by an attack of livers wind to the face. Patients may suffer from high irritability, anger, distension, and pain in both costal regions, belching, sighing.

- **Treatment**

1. Foot meridian acupuncture:
BL-67 (Zhiyin 至阴), ST-45 (Lidui 厉兑), GB 43 (Xiaxi 侠溪), GB-44 (Zuqiaoyin 足窍阴)

2. Foot acupuncture: Face, Head and face, Heart, Liver

3. Foot massage: Trigeminal nerve, Head, Liver, Heart, Spleen, Kidney, Stomach

I-14 Facial Paralysis 面瘫 Miantan
Deviation of Eye and Mouth 口眼歪斜
Kouyanwaixie

This is a condition caused by the inflammation of facial nerves. Deviated mouth and eyes are the common name. The paralysis appears mostly on one side, mostly among young and middle-aged people.

- **Differentiation**

This is caused by weakness of the channels, which are attacked by the exogenous pathogenic wind-cold or wind-heat and led to the flaccidness of muscles by Qi stagnation and blood stasis in the channels of face.

- **Treatment**

1. Foot meridian acupuncture:
BL-67 (Zhiyin 至阴), ST-45 (Lidui 厉兑), GB-43 (Xiaxi 侠溪), GB-44 (Zuqiaoyin 足窍阴)

2. Foot acupuncture: Face, Head and face, Heart, Liver

3. Foot massage: Trigeminal nerve, Head, Ear, Frontal sinus, Liver, Spleen, Kidney, Eye

I-15 Sunstroke 中暑 Zhongshu

It is due to strong sunlight or staying in high temperature time. It mostly happens among elderly and weak people.

- **Differentiation**
1. Mild type
The main manifestations are headache, fever, flushed face, nausea, fatigue, irritability, thirst, rapid thready pulse.

2. Severe type
The main manifestations are headache, high fever, thirst, short breathing, loss of consciousness, sweating, suddenly collapse, deep, forceless pulse.

- **Treatment**
1. Foot meridian acupuncture:

ST-41 (Jiexi 解溪), ST-44 (Neiting 内庭), KI-1 (Yongquan 涌泉), BL-66 (Zutonggu 足通谷), EX (Zuxin), EX (Dazhi Jumao), EX (Xiaozhijian), EX (Qiduan)

I-16 Hypertension 高血压 Gaoxueya

This is caused by excessive liver fire. Patients may suffer from headache, vertigo, flushed face, red eyes.

- **Treatment**
1. Foot meridian acupuncture:
ST-41 (Jiexi 解溪), Liv-31 (Taichong 太冲), Liv-2 (Xingjian 行间), BL-60 (Kunlun 昆仑), BL-62 (Shenmai 申脉), GB-43 (Xiaxi 侠溪), KI-6 (Zhaohai 照海), GB-44 (Zuqiaoyin 足窍阴), ST-41 (Jiexi 解溪), KI-4 (Dazhong 大钟), EX (Dazhi Jumao), EX (Xiaozhijian tip of the little toe), EX (Zuxin)

2. Foot acupuncture: Heart, Kidney, Vertigo
3. Foot massage: Head, Brain stem and cerebellum, Kidney, Liver, Gallbladder, Heart, Urinary bladder, Balance organ (Labyrinth)

I-17 Hemiplegia 偏瘫 Piantan

It is a condition which includes impairment of movement or paralysis of the limbs on one side. It is mostly seen among the aged people with a history of hypertension and arteriosclerosis.

- **Treatment**
1. Foot meridian acupuncture:
ST-41(Jiexi 解溪), ST-45 (Lidui 厉兑), GB-40 (Qiuxu 丘墟), BL-60 (Kunlun 昆仑), BL-61 (Pucan 仆参), BL-62 (Shenmai 申脉), KI-1 (Yongquan 涌泉), EX (Xiakunlun), EX (Dazhi Jumao)
2. Foot massage: Head, Frontal sinus, Brain stem and Cerebellum, Shoulder, Hip joint, Pituitary gland, Adrenal gland, Kidney, Heart, Spleen, Knee, Elbow joint

I-18 Palpitation 心悸 Xinji

- **Differentiation**
1. Qi and Blood Insufficiency
The manifestations are lassitude, palpitation, pallor, disturbed sleep, pale tongue, weak thready pulse.

2. Phlegm-Fire Disturbance
The manifestations are restlessness, dream-disturbed sleep, irritability, yellow urine, sticky sputum, yellow greasy tongue coating, rapid slippery pulse.

2. Blood Status
The manifestations are sallow emaciated complexion, palpitation, asthmatic breathing, cold limbs, thready, choppy pulse.

- **Treatment**

1. Foot meridian acupuncture:
GB-41 (Zulinqi 足临泣), BL-62 (Shenmai 申脉), BL-64 (Jinggu 京骨), SP-3 (Taibai 太白), KI-2 (Rangu 然谷), ST-43 (Xiangu 陷谷), ST-44 (Neiting 内庭)

2. Foot acupuncture: Heart, Heart pain, EX (Neizhiyin)
3. Foot massage: Heart, Kidney, Spleen, Head, Thyroid gland, Adrenal gland

I-19 Hysteria 脏躁 Zangzao

This is a neurological condition involving psychological syndromes caused by mental depression and mental distress due to the stagnation of Qi.

- **Differentiation**

1. Liver Qi Stagnation
This type is characterized by restlessness, mental depression, poor self-control, irritability, red tongue coating, wiry pulse.

2. Emotional Depression
This type is characterized by low spirit, emotional unrest, constant cries with grief or sorrow, pale tongue with white coating, thready pulse.

- **Treatment**

1. Foot meridian acupuncture:
Liv-2 (Xingjian 行间), Liv-3 (Taichong 太冲), EX (Neizhiyin), EX (Nuxi)
2. Foot acupuncture: Epilepsy, Anmian, Liver
3. Foot massage: Pituitary gland, Spleen, Stomach, Liver, Kidney, Heart, Lung

I-20 Hiccups 呃逆 Eni

- **Differentiation**
1. Retention of food and stagnation of Qi
Epigastric and abdominal distension, sticky, yellow tongue coating, rolling forceful pulse.

2. Attack by pathogenic Cold
Alleviated by hot drinks, white moist tongue coating, slow pulse.

- **Treatment**
1. Foot massage: Coeliac plexus, parathyroid gland, diaphragm, stomach, kidney, duodenum

I-21 Impotence 阳痿 Yangwei

- **Differentiation**
It is characterized by the penis inability and erection. The manifestation shows, dizziness, blurring vision, listlessness, poor sprit, frequent urination, weakness knee and lumbar region, insomnia, palpitation, Heart and Spleen may be involved.

- **Treatment**
1. Foot massage:

Reproductive gland, penis, inguinal groove, pituitar gland, prostate gland, adrenal gland, kidney reflecting area.

I-22 Insomnia 不寐 Bumei

- **Differentiation**

1. Heart and Spleen Deficiency

Difficulty in falling asleep and disturbed sleep, palpitation, poor memory, poor appetite, loose stool, sallow complexion, thin white tongue coating, thready weak pulse.

2.Heart and Kidney Disharmony

Insomnia accompanied by dizziness, tinnitus, leukorrhagia, feverish sensation in the palms and soles, red tongue with less coating, rapid weak pulse.

3.Liver Fire Disturbance

Manifestations are dizziness, short temper, restlessness, hypochondriac pain, thin yellow tongue, wiry rapid pulse.

4.Stomach Dysfunction

Insomnia accompanied by fullness in the epigastric region, abdominal distension, belching, acid regurgitation, yellow greasy tongue coating, wiry pulse.

- **Treatment**
1. Foot meridian acupuncture:
BL-62 (Shenmai 申脉), KI-6 (Zhaohai 照海), Liv-2 (Xingjian 行间), Liv-3 (Taichong 太冲), EX (Insomnia), EX (Zuxin), tip of little toe (Xiaozhijian)

2. Foot acupuncture:
Anmian, Heart, Stomach, Spleen
3. Foot massage:
Frontal sinus, Parathyroid gland, Head, Brain stem and Cerebellum, Thyroid gland, Spleen, Kidney

I-23 Incontinence of urine 尿失禁 Niaoshijin
This is the involuntary discharge of urine.

- **Treatment**
   1. Foot meridian acupuncture:

KI-1 (Yongquan 涌泉), GB-41 (Zulinqi 足临泣), KI-3 (Taixi 太溪), Liv-3 (Taichong 太冲), Liv-4 (Zhongfeng 中风)

2. Foot acupuncture: Bladder, Kidney

3. Foot massage: Kidney, Urinary bladder, Ureter, Prostate gland, Urethra and Pituitary gland

I-24 Lumbago 腰痛 Yaotong

The symptoms are pain in the waist area. This is the diseases of spinal column, injury of soft tissues beside spinal column, compression of spinal nerve roots or gynecological diseases.

- **Treatment**

1. Foot meridian acupuncture:

ST-41 (Jiexi 解溪), KI-1 (Yongquan 涌泉), KI-3 (Taixi 太溪), KI-4 (Dazhong 大钟), Liv-3 (Taichong 太冲), BL-65 (Shugu 束骨), EX (Xiakunlun 下昆仑), EX (Quanshengzu)

2. Foot acupuncture: Lumbago, waist and leg, kidney ischium

3. Foot massage: Kidney, Lumbar spine, Ureter, Urinary bladder

I-25 Nephritis 肾炎 Shenyan

This is caused by the invasion of external pathogens and dysfunction of lung, spleen and kidney. The patient may suffer from edema, hypertension, hematuria, and proteinuria.

- **Treatment**
1. Foot meridian acupuncture:
ST-41 (Jiexi 解溪), ST-43 (Xiangu 陷谷), SP-3 (Taibai 太白), KI-3 (Taixi 太溪), KI-5 (Shuiquan 水泉), Liv 2 (Xingjian 行间), Liv-3 (Taichong 太冲)
2. Foot acupuncture: Kidney, Spleen, Bladder, Liver
3. Foot massage: Kidney, Ureter, Urinary bladder, Spleen, Liver, Lung, Lymph nodes, Adrenal gland

I-26 Obesity 肥胖 Feipang

It refers to excessive accumulation of fat in the body tissues. Clinically, it is divided into Simple and Secondary types.
Simple Obesity: It is due to overeating of greasy, sweet food that exceeds the normal consumption of body heat.

Secondary Obesity: It is caused by hypothalamic pituitary lesions and over-secretion of hydrocortisone.

- **Manifestations**

Patients have visible fat accumulations in the neck, lower abdomen, and buttock. Mild obese patients do not have signs of symptom, but severe patients have metabolic disturbances of aversion to heat, profuse sweating, fatigue, dizziness, headache, palpitation.

- **Treatment**

1. Foot meridian acupuncture:

ST-41 (Jiexi 解溪), ST-44 (Neiting 内庭), ST-43 (Xiangu 陷谷), SP-4 (Gongsun 公孙), SP-5 (Shangqiu 商丘), SP-3 (Taibai 太白), SP-1 (Yinbai 隐白), KI-3 (Taixi 太溪), Liv-1 (Dadun 大敦), Liv-3 (Taichong 太冲)

2. Foot massage: Spleen, Stomach, Kidney, Lower abdomen, Thyroid gland, Pituitary gland

I-27 Psychosis 精神病 Jingshenbing

There is divided into two types.

1) It is characterized by an apathetic expression, silence, mental dullness, speaking nonsense, and diminished motion.

2) It is characterized by mental excitement, hyper-irritability, restlessness, noise making, beating and scolding others, destruction and extreme fury.

- **Treatment**
1. Foot meridian acupuncture:
BL-61 (Pucan 仆参), BL-66 (Zutonggu 足通谷), SP-5 (Shangqiu 商丘), KI-6 (Zhaohai 照海), BL-62 (Shenmai 申脉), EX (Nuxi)
2. Foot acupuncture: Anmian, Kidney, Liver, Heart

3. Foot massage: Head, Pituitary gland, Thyroid gland, Spleen, Heart, Liver, Kidney

I-28 Ptosis of stomach 胃下垂 Weixiachui

This is a condition that the stomach is at an abnormally low position. It is characterized of Liver Qi stagnation, from anger, mental depression, aggravation of symptoms after emotional disturbance.

- **Treatment**

1. Foot meridian acupuncture:
ST-42 (Chongyang 冲阳), SP-5 (Shangqiu 商丘), ST-44 (Neiting 内庭), SP-1 (Yinbai 隐白), Liv-3 (Taichong 太冲)

2. Foot acupuncture: Stomach, spleen, stomach and intestine

3. Foot massage: Stomach, Kidney, Duodenum, Small intestine, Colon (ascend, transverse, descend)

I-29 Poor memory 记忆力差 Jiyilicha

- **Differentiation**

1. Heart and Spleen Deficiency
It includes forgetfulness, weakness of limbs, palpitation, poor sleep, pallor complexion, pale tongue, thin white greasy tongue coating, weak thready pulse.

2. Heart and Kidney Disharmony

It includes forgetfulness, lumbar soreness, tinnitus, sensation in the palms and soles, restlessness, poor sleep, red tongue, thin rapid pulse.

3. Poor Sprit
It involves aging. The manifestations ae forgetfulness, poor appetite, lumbar soreness, frequent urination, palpitation, poor sleep, thin white tongue coating, weak thready pulse.

4.Phlegm-Fluid Status
The manifestations are forgetfulness, low speech, white greasy tongue coating, thin rapid pulse.

• **Treatment**
1. Foot meridian acupuncture:
BL-60 (Kunlun 昆仑), BL-61 (Pucan 仆参), KI-3 (Taixi 太溪), SP-3 (Taibai 太白), SP-5 (Shangqiu 商丘), KI-2 (Rangu 然谷)
2. Foot massage: Head, Brain stem and cerebellum, Thyroid gland, Adrenal gland, Pituitary gland, Spleen, Kidney, Heart

I-30 Shoulder Pain 肩痛 Jiantong

Shoulder pain is named in TCM as frozen shoulder or fifty years old shoulder. The exogenous pathogenic wind, cold and damp overcome patients who are exhausted, overstrained, injured, and while sleeping in the shoulder.

- **Differentiation**

Pain on shoulders alleviates in the daytime and worsens at night. It may involve back. It may aggravate with cold and alleviate with warmth.

- **Treatment**
    1. Foot meridian acupuncture:
    BL.60 (Kunlun 昆仑), BL-64 (Jinggu 京骨), ST-45 (Lidui 厉兑), GB-40 (Qiuxu 丘墟)
    2. Foot acupuncture: Ischium

I-31 Rheumatoid Arthritis 类风湿关节炎 Reifengshiguanjieyan

This is a kind of chronic and immune.

- **Differentiation**

The manifestations are swelling, stiffness, deformity of the joints, pain. It involves wrist, elbow, knee shoulder, ankle.

1. Cold-Damp
2. Damp-Heat

- **Treatment**

1. Foot meridian acupuncture:
ST-42 (Chongyang 冲阳), ST-43 (Xiangu 陷谷), GB-40 (Qiuxu 丘墟), GB-41 (Zulinqi 足临泣), GB-42 (Diwuhui 地五会), BL-61 (Pucan 仆参), BL-63 (Jinmen 金门), SP-5 (Shangqiu 商丘)
2. Foot massage: Thoracic spine, Lumbar spine, Kidney, Spleen, Lung, Hip joint, Knee, Elbow joint

I-32 Retention of urine 癃闭 Longbi

- **Differentiation**

1. Accumulation of Damp-Heat in the Urinary Bladder
The manifestations are distention in the lower abdomen, hot scanty urine, thirst but no desire to drink, red tongue with yellow coating, rapid pulse.

2. Kidney-Qi Deficient
The manifestations are dribbling of urine, lumbar soreness, listlessness, pallor complexion,

weakness of knee, pale tongue, deep thready pulse.

3.Urethral Obstruction
The manifestations are dribbling of urine, pain and distention in lower abdomen, red spot on the tongue, rapid pulse.

- **Treatment**
1. Foot meridian acupuncture:
KI-4 (Dazhong 大钟), KI-5 (Shuiquan 水泉), Liv-3 (Taichong 太冲), KI-1 (Yongquan 涌泉), BL-67 (Zhiyin 至阴)
2. Foot acupuncture: Uterus, Bladder, Kidney, Spleen, Lung
3. Foot massage: Lung, Spleen, Kidney, Liver, Urinary bladder, Ureter, Urethra, Prostate gland

I-33 Abdominal Pain 腹痛 Futong

- **Differentiation**
1. Internal accumulation of cold:
Sudden violent pain which responds to warmth and is aggravated by cold. Other manifestations include loose stools, profuse clear urine, white coated tongue, deep tense or deep slow pulse.

2. Retention of food:
Epigastric and abdominal distension and pain which may be aggravated by pressure, foul belching and acidity. Abdominal pain may be accompanied by diarrhea and relieved after defecation. The tongue is sticky coated, the pulse is rolling.

- **Treatment**
1. Foot meridian acupuncture:
SP-4 (Gongsun 公孙), SP-2 (Dadu 大都), SP-3 (Taibai 太白), Liv-2 (Xingjian 行间), BL-67 (Zhiyin 至阴)
2. Foot acupuncture: Stomach, Stomach and Intestine, Spleen, Small Intestine
3. Foot massage: Stomach, Duodenum, Spleen, Lymph nodes, Coeliac plexus

I-34 Stranguria 排尿困难 Painiaokunnan

It is characterized by frequent urination with pain in urethra and sensation of unfinished urination. Patients with stranguria of the heat type may suffer from dysuria with frequent discharge of small amount of dark, turbid urine and burning pain in urethra, distending sensation in lower abdomen.

- **Treatment**
1. Foot meridian acupuncture:
KI-3 (Taixi 太溪)
2. Foot acupuncture: Bladder, Kidney, Bed-wetting
3. Foot massage: Kidney, Urinary bladder, Ureter, Parathyroid gland, Lymph nodes (abdomen), Stomach, Lung, Prostate gland

I-35 Sciatica 坐骨神经 Zuogushenjingtong

This is the pain radiating to the sciatic nerve distribution in the hip region, posterior lateral aspect of the leg.

- **Manifestations**
1. Primary Sciatica
It is characterized by a sudden onset of continuous sharp pain, worsens with cold, alleviates with warmth.

2. Secondary Sciatica
This is a slow onset of pain which may involve primary lesions, radiating pain due to lumbar

disc degeneration. The pain is worse with cough, sneezing.

- **Treatment**

1. Foot meridian acupuncture:
BL-60 (Kunlun 昆仑), BL-61 (Pucan 仆参), BL-62 (Shenmai 申脉), BL-63 (Jinmen 金门), BL-65 (Shugu 束谷)
2. Foot acupuncture: Buttocks, Waist and Leg, Ischium 1, Ischium 2
3. Foot massage: Sciatic nerve, Lumbar spine, Sacrum, Knee, Kidney, Spleen

I-36 Stiff Neck 落枕 Laozhen

- **Differentiation**

It is caused by exogenous pathogenic wind, cold and while sleeping. Some cases may have the pain spread to the shoulder of the affected side, and it aggravate by movement of the neck.

- **Treatment**

1. Foot meridian acupuncture:

BL-64 (Jinggu 京骨), BL-65 (Shugu 束谷), BL-60 (Kunlun 昆仑), GB-40 (Qiuxu 丘墟), ST-45 (Lidui 厉兑)

2. Foot acupuncture:
 Stiff neck

3. Foot massage:
Neck, Cervical spine, Trapezius muscle, Kidney

I-37 Vomiting 呕吐 Outu

- **Differentiation**

1. Retention of Food
This is characterized by epigastric distention, casting up of sour tastes, belching, abdominal pain, foul gas, constipation, greasy tongue coating, slippery pulse.

2. Invasion of Stomach by Liver Qi
This is characterized by vomiting, acid regurgitation, frequent belching, distention in the hypochondriac region, thin greasy tongue coating, wiry pulse.

3. Weakness of Stomach and Spleen

Sallow complexion, lack of appetite, loose stools, pale, sticky tongue, weak soft pulse.

- **Treatment**
1. Foot meridian acupuncture:
GB-40 (Qiuxu 丘墟), BL-61 (Pucan 仆参), BL-66 (Zutonggu 足通谷), SP-1 (Yinbai 隐白), SP-2 (Dadu 大都), SP-3 (Taibai 太白)
2. Foot acupuncture:
Stomach, Colon, Small Intestine, Spleen
3. Foot massage:
Spleen, Stomach, Coeliac plexus, Liver, Duodenum

I-38 Dizziness 眩晕 Xuanyun

- **Differentiation**
1. Hyperactivity of Liver Yang
The manifestations are tinnitus, nausea, backache disturbed sleep, flushed face, congested eyes, red tongue proper with thin yellow coating, wiry rapid pulse.

2. Qi and Blood Deficiency

The manifestations are palpitation, insomnia, pale complexion, pale complexion, poor appetite, pale tongue proper, weak pulse.

3. Phlegm-Damp obstruction in the interior
The manifestations are lassitude, fullness in the chest and epigastrium, heaviness of head, vomiting, white and sticky tongue, rolling pulse.

- **Treatment**
1. Foot meridian acupuncture:
BL-60 (Kunlun 昆仑), BL-62 (Shenmai 申脉), Liv-2 (Xingjian 行间), Liv-3 (Taichong 太冲), ST-41 (Jiexi 解溪), EX (Dazhi Jumao)

2. Foot acupuncture:
Kidney, Vertigo, Liver, Lung, Spleen
3. Foot massage:
Head, Brain stem and cerebellum, Pituitary gland, Balance organ (labyrinth), Frontal sinus, Kidney

II. Gynecology

II-1 Amenorrhea 闭经 Bijing

- **Differentiation**

1. Blood Stasis
This type of Amenorrhea is characterized by an absence of menses, distention and pain in the lower abdomen, aggravated by pressing, but relieved by warmth, purplish dark tongue, deep wiry pulse.

2. Blood Deficiency
This type of Amenorrhea is characterized by delayed menstrual period, and gradually decreasing in amount of flow. It is accompanied by soreness in the lumbar region and knees, dizziness, loose stool, palpitation, pale, white coating tongue, thready, weak pulse.

- **Treatment**

1. Foot meridian acupuncture:
GB-43 (Xiaxi 侠溪), KI-5 (Shuiquan 水泉), Liv-1 (Dadun 大敦), Liv-2 (Xingjian 行间)

2. Foot massage: Pituitary gland, Kidney, Reproductive gland, Thyroid gland, Coeliac plexus, Adrenal gland

II-2 Malposition of Fetus 胎位不正 Taiweibuzheng

- **Differentiation**

Malposition of Fetus means that the fetus is in an abnormal position in the uterus after thirty weeks of pregnancy. It is often seen in multipara or pregnant women who have laxity of the abdominal wall.

- **Treatment**

1. Foot meridian acupuncture:
BL-67 (Zhiyin 至阴)
2. Foot massage: Kidney, Reproductive gland, Uterus, Adrenal gland, Pituitary gland

II-3 Dysmenorrhea 痛经 Tongjing

- **Differentiation**

1. Status of Qi and Blood

This type is premenstrual cramping pain fixed in the lower abdomen.

Distending pain of lower abdomen with distention in the breast and the hypochondriac region which appears before or after menstrual flow, accompanied by dripping of scanty dark purplish in color with clots, dark purplish tongue, wiry pulse.

2. Liver and Kidney Yin Deficiency

This type of lower abdominal pain at late stage of menstruation or post menstruation, and relieved by pressing during or post the menstrual flow. It is mild pain but persistent pain. The scanty flow and pink in color, may be accompanied by dizziness, palpitation, soreness in the lumbar region and knees, thin white tongue coating, deep thready pulse.

- **Treatment**

1. Foot meridian acupuncture:

ST-44 (Neiting 内庭), GB-44 (Zuqiaoyin 足窍阴), KI-5 (Shuiquan 水泉), EX (Quchi 曲池)

2. Foot acupuncture:

Uterus, Dysmenorrhea 2

3. Foot massage:

Kidney, pituitary gland, Reproductive gland, Inguinal groove, Lower abdomen

II-4 Hypogalactia 缺乳 Qiuru

This is a condition where excretion of milk in nursing mothers who is insufficient. It occurs in mothers with deficiency of Qi and blood, sallow complexion, dizziness, poor appetite.

- **Treatment**
1. Foot meridian acupuncture:
Liv-3 (Taichong 太冲), GB-42 (Diwuhui 地五会)
2. Foot massage:
Lymph nodes (upper body), Pituitary gland, Parathyroid gland, Kidney, Adrenal gland, chest, Reproductive gland, Lymph nodes

II-5 Hyperplasia of Breast 乳腺增生 Ruxianzengsheng

This is a disease of older women who have breast masses caused by stagnation of Liv-Qi or accumulation of phlegm and dampness.

- **Treatment**
1. Foot meridian acupuncture:
GB-41 (Zulinqi), GB-42 (Diwuhui, Liv-3 (Taichong)
2. Foot acupuncture: Lung
3. Foot massage: Chest, Lymph nodes (chest), Lymph nodes (upper body), Lymph nodes (abdomen), Kidney, Ureter, Urinary bladder, Reproductive gland

II-6 Irregular Menstruation 月经不调 Yuejingbutiao

- **Differentiation**
1. Precede Menstrual Flow
The flow is advanced at least more than seven days, and it may appear fresh red or purple red color. The symptoms appear irritability, dry mouth, night sweating, feverish palms and soles, red tongue with less coating, rapid thready pulse.

2. Delayed Menstrual Flow
This condition may the type of deficiency or excess factors. Deficiency caused by deficiency

nutrient blood or Yang Qi. Excess caused by stagnation of Qi and Blood of Chong and Ren Channels, which leads to delayed menstrual flow.

3. Disorder of Menstrual Flow

This condition is mostly caused by impaired circulation of Qi and Blood due to stagnation of Liver Qi, deficiency of Kidney Qi, and the factors are such as emotional depression, anger, as a result, it become disorderly menstrual flow.

- **Treatment**

1. Foot meridian acupuncture:

Liv-3 (Taichong 太冲), KI-3 (Taixi 太溪), KI-2 (Rangu 然谷), SP-1 (Yinbai 隐白), EX (duyin), EX Yingchi, EX (Tongli)

2. Foot acupuncture: Uterus, Dysmenorrhea 1, Dysmenorrhea 2

3. Foot massage: Pituitary gland, Kidney, Reproductive gland, Uterus, Lower abdomen, Adrenal gland, Thyroid gland, Coeliac plexus

II-7 Infertility 不孕症 Buyunzheng

- **Differentiation**

1. Kidney Deficiency
It relates to irregular menstruations, and scanty flow of light red color. The manifestations are tinnitus, dizziness, soreness of lumbar region and knee, pale white tongue coating, and deep thready pulse.

2. Blood Deficiency
It relates to scanty flow light red color, and delayed menstruation. The manifestations are emaciation, dizziness, lassitude, pale tongue with little coating, deep thready pulse.

3. Cold in Uterus
It relates to have normal menstruation, but its cycle is sometimes prolonged with dark clots. The manifestations are cold limbs, pain in the lower abdomen, profuse urine, pale tongue with white coating, and deep slow pulse.

4. Phlegm-Damp Retention
It relates an obese constitution, prolonged cycle, profuse sticky leukorrhea, dizziness, palpitation, white sticky tongue coating, and soft, slippery pulse.

- **Treatment**

1. Foot meridian acupuncture:
KI-1 (Yongquan 涌泉), KI-2 (Rangu 然谷)
2. Foot massage: Pituitary gland, Kidney, Reproductive gland, Uterus, Vagina, Thyroid gland, Parathyroid gland, Adrenal gland, Ureter, Urinary bladder

II-8 Leukorrhagia 带下 Daixia

- **Differentiation**

Leukorrhea may be differentiated as white or yellow discharge.

1. Spleen Deficiency
White or slight yellowish of sticky quality without foul smell. The manifestations are loose stool, sallow complexion, lassitude, pale tongue with sticky coating, and slow weak pulse.

2. Kidney Deficiency
It may be much white and dilute quality discharge, accompanied by soreness in the lumbar region, loose stool, frequent urination, pale tongue with white coating, and deep slow pulse.

3. Damp-Heat Retention

It is yellow discharge with bad odor, and accompanied by itching in the virgina, scanty urination, thirst, sticky yellow tongue, and rapid slippery pulse.

- **Treatment**

1. Foot meridian acupuncture
SP-1 (Yinbai 隐白), Liv-2 (Xingjian 行间), EX (Yingchi), EX (Yinyang)
2. Foot acupuncture: Uterus, Dysmenorrhea1, Dysmenorrhea 2
3. Foot massage: Uterus, Vagina, Kidney

II-9 Mastitis 乳腺炎 Ruxianyan

This is infection of the breast during the breast-feeding period, and often in the upper and lateral quarter of one breast.

- **Treatment**

1. Foot meridian acupuncture:
GB-41 (Zulinqi 足临泣), GB-42 (Diwuhui 地五会), KI-6 (Zhaohai 照海), GB-43 (Xiaxi 侠溪), BL-65 (Shugu 束骨), Liv-2 (Xingjian 行间), Liv-3 (Taichong 太冲)

2. Foot acupuncture: Lung

II-10 Menopause 绝经 Juejing

It is usually seen in woman who is about 55 years old, and at the period before or after termination.

- **Manifestation**

The manifestations are sudden termination or disorder of menstruation, and flushed face, lassitude, sweating, listlessness, depression, irritability, insomnia, palpitation.

- **Treatment**

1. Foot meridian acupuncture:
Liv-3 (Taichong 太冲) KI-3 (Taixi 太溪), KI-6 (Zhaohai 照海)
2. Foot massage: Head, Neck, Adrenal gland, Pituitary gland, Uterus, Reproductive gland, thyroid gland, Pancreas, Coeliac plexus

II-11 Postpartum fainting 产后昏厥 Chanhou hunjue

This occurs after childbirth with dizziness, vertigo, nausea, vomiting restlessness.

- **Treatment**
  1. Foot meridian acupuncture:
  KI-1 (Yongquan 涌泉), KI-2 (Rangu 然谷), KI-6 (Zhaohai 照海), Liv-2 (Xingjian 行间), EX (Dazhi Jumao)
  2. Foot acupuncture: Vertigo, Kidney
  3. Foot massage: Kidney, Heart, Spleen, Ureter, Adrenal gland

II-12 Prolapse of uterus 子宫脱垂 Zigong tuochui

This is usually appearing after childbirth. It is characterized by spastic sensation in lower abdomen, weakness of limbs, shallow breath, no desire to speak sallow complexion, deficiency of kidney.

- **Treatment**

1. Foot meridian acupuncture: KI-5 (Shuiquan 水泉)
2. Foot massage: Uterus, Vagina

II-13 Pudendal itching 阴部瘙痒 Yinbu saoyang

This is an intractable itching in the perineal region and vagina, radiated to medial side of thigh. It is characterized by restlessness, profuse discharge of leukorrhea, annoyance.

- **Treatment**
1. Foot meridian acupuncture:
KI-6 (Zhaohai 照海), KI-2 (Rangu 然谷)
2. Foot massage: Kidney, Ureter, Urinary bladder, Adrenal gland, Uterus, Reproductive gland, Vagina

II-14 Pregnancy vomiting 怀孕呕吐 Huaiyunoutu

It is characterized by nausea, vomiting, dizziness, anorexia, distension of upper abdomen, nausea, vomiting, mental fatigue, sleepiness.

- **Treatment**

1. Foot meridian acupuncture:
ST-44 (Neiting 内庭), GB-44 (Qiuxu 丘墟), Liv-3 (Taichong 太冲), SP-4 (Gongsun 公孙), Ex (Duyin), EX (Neihuai Qianxia), EX (Nuxi)

2. Foot acupuncture: Stomach
3. Foot massage: Pituitary gland, Kidney, Ureter, Urinary bladder, Thyroid gland, Adrenal gland, Uterus

III. Pediatric Diseases

III-1 Infantile Convulsion 小儿惊风 Xiaoerjingfeng

Infants are not physically developed, and they are mentally weak. This is a common acute disease that may include coma, convulsions of limbs, lockjaw.

- **Differentiation**

1. Acute Convulsion

The manifestations are high fever, clenched jaws, upward staring eyes, contraction, rattles, rapid and wiry pulse.

2. Chronic Convulsion

The manifestations are pallor, lassitude, emaciation, intermittent convulsion, loose stools, clear urine, weak pulse.

- **Treatment**

1. Foot meridian acupuncture:

KI-1 (Yongquan 涌泉), Liv-3 (Taichong 太冲), GB-44 (Zuqiaoyin 足窍阴), EX (Neizhiyin), EX (Lineiting)

2. Foot massage: Head, Adrenal gland, Pituitary gland, Parathyroid gland, Tonsil, Spleen, Lymph nodes

III-2 Enuresis 遗尿症 Yiniaozheng

It refers to involuntary discharge of the urine of a child. It happens to occur during sleep.

- **Differentiation**

It may be happened in several nights during sleep. The manifestations are listlessness, poor appetite.

- **Treatment**

1. Foot meridian acupuncture:
Liv-3 (Taichong 太冲), Liv-2 (Xingjian 行间), KI-5 (Shuiquan 水泉), KI-3 (Taixi 太溪)
2. Foot acupuncture: Bed-wetting
3. Foot massage: Kidney, Ureter, Urinary bladder, Urethra, Pituitary gland

III-3 Infantile Diarrhea 小儿腹泻 Xiaoerfuxie

It is a common pediatric disease, mainly manifested by frequent bowel movement, watery feces. It may occur in any season, but more often occurs in summer and autumn.

- **Differentiation**

1. Cold-Damp
The stool is watery, abdominal pain, accompanied by aversion to cold, pale tongue with thin coating, and thin deep pulse.

2. Damp-Heat

The manifestations are the yellowish stool, watery, feverish sensation, yellow and greasy tongue coating, slippery rapid pulse.

3. Food Retention

The manifestations are epigastric distension that alleviated by bowel movement, poor appetite, vomiting, thick yellow greasy tongue coating, full slippery pulse.

4. Yang Deficiency

It characterized by watery stool, cold limbs, poor spirit, pale tongue with white coating, and thready pulse.

- **Treatment**

1. Foot meridian acupuncture:
SP-3 (Taibai 太白), SP-4 (Gongsun 公孙), EX (Yinyang), EX (Nuxi)
2. Foot acupuncture: Spleen, small intestine, Colon
3. Foot massage: Coeliac plexus, small intestine, Stomach, Colon, Duodenum, Liver, Gallbladder, Spleen

III-4 Epidemic parotitis (mumps)流行性腮腺炎 Liuxingsingsaixianyan)

This is an acute infectious disease characterized by painful swelling of the parotidean region caused by epidemic pathogenic wind.

- **Differentiation**
1. Pathogenic Heat invading the Exterior
The manifestations are slight fever with aversion to cold, slight yellowish tongue coating, and rapid superficial pulse.

2. Pathogenic Heat Accumulation
The manifestations are pain, feverish sensation, aggravated by pressing, high fever, headache, vomiting, constipation, straw urine, pain and swelling in the testis, red tongue with yellow coating, and rapid superficial pulse.

- **Treatment**
1. Foot meridian acupuncture:
SP-2 (Dadu 大都), ST-43 (Xiangu 陷谷), ST-44 (Neiting 内庭), KI-2 (Rangu 然谷)
2. Foot acupuncture: Tonsil 1, Tonsil 2, Vertigo

3. Foot massage: Pituitary gland, Adrenal gland, Lymph nodes (upper body), Larynx, Tonsil

III-5 Infantile Malnutrition 小儿营养不良 Yingyangbuliang

It is found more often in children under five years old. It is related to the factors of irregular food intake, lactation, parasite diseases, weaken of Qi and Blood, Spleen and Stomach.

- **Differentiation**

It is characterized by emaciation, listlessness, sallow complexion, loose muscles.
It is accompanied by poor appetite, poor sleep, loose watery stool, pale tongue, and weak thready pulse.

- **Treatment**

1. Foot meridian acupuncture:
ST-44 (Neiting 内庭), SP-4 (Gongsun 公孙), SP-5 (Shangqiu 商丘), EX (Ranhou)
2. Foot acupuncture: Stomach and Spleen

3. Foot massage: Stomach, Duodenum, Liver, Gallbladder, small intestine, Spleen, Coeliac plexus

III-6 Whooping Cough 百日咳 Bairike

It is one of the common respiratory infectious diseases, which the seasonal epidemic invasions that produce turbid phlegm in the interior of the body.

- **Differentiation**

1. First stage

The manifestations are cough, aversion to cold with fever, loss of voice, thin white tongue coating, and superficial pulse.

2. Second stage

Wheezing sounds in the throat, feels better in the daytime, difficult in the night, straw urine, constipation, yellow tongue coating, and slippery rapid pulse.

3. Recovering stage

Less cough day by day, spontaneous sweating, hoarseness of voice, red tongue with thin, and thready rapid pulse.

- **Treatment**

1. Foot meridian acupuncture:
GB-44 (Zuqiaoyin 足窍阴), KI-4 (Dazhong 大钟)
2. Foot acupuncture: Lung
3. Foot massage: Pituitary gland, Lung, Adrenal gland, Kidney, Lymph nodes (upper body)

III-7 Poliomyelitis 脊髓灰质炎 Jisuihuizhiyan

This is an acute epidemic disease caused by the poliomyelitis virus. This is caused by an attack of wind, dampness and heat pathogens through the mouth to the lungs and stomach. At the early stage, there are fever, cough, red throat, vomiting and diarrhea. There will also be pain in limbs, numbness, and paralysis of the limbs.

- **Treatment**
1. Foot meridian acupuncture:
ST-41 (Jiexi 解溪), ST-42 (Chongyang 冲阳), ST-44 (Neiting 内庭), ST-45 (Lidui 厉兑), EX (Xiakunlun 下昆仑)
2. Foot massage: Pituitary gland, Head, Cerebellum, Coeliac plexus, Lymph nodes (upper body), Lymph nodes (abdomen), Stomach, small intestine, Liver, Gallbladder

IV. Surgical and Dermatological Disease

IV-1 Alopecia 脱发症 Tuofazheng

This is the scalp with loss of hair in localized areas. The hair may be suddenly lost overnight in a single or multiple areas.

- **Differentiation**

It may be caused by mental stress, anxiety, sudden nervous shock.
(1) Liver and Kidney Yin Deficiency

- **Treatment**
1. Foot meridian acupuncture:
SP-4 (Gongsun 公孙), KI-3 (Taixi 太溪)

2. Foot acupuncture:
 Head and face, Anmian, Lung, Kidney
3. Foot massage: Kidney, Lung, Head, Pituitary gland, Parathyroid gland, Adrenal gland, Ureter, Urinary bladder, Reproductive gland

IV-2 Cholecystitis 胆囊炎 Dannangyan

This is infection of the gallbladder caused by bacterial infection and bile stasis.
- **Treatment**
1. Foot meridian acupuncture:
GB-44 (Zuqiaoyin 足窍阴), GB-42 (Diwuhui 地五会), GB-41 (Zulinqi 足临泣), EX (Quchi)
2. Foot acupuncture: Liver

IV-3 Constrictive tenosynovitis 缩窄性腱鞘炎 Suozhaixingjianqiaoyan

This is caused by chronic strain of the fingers and wrist related to the job. It causes edema, and the movement of the tendons may be impaired.

- **Treatment**
1. Foot meridian acupuncture: BL-60 (Kunlun 昆仑), BL-65 (Shugu 束谷), GB-42 (Diwuhui 地五会), BL-62 (Shenmai 申脉), KI-1 (Yongquan 涌泉), KI-3 (Taixi 太溪), Liv-2 (Xingjian 行间), GB-40 (Qiuxu 丘墟), EX (Xiakunlun, EX (Quanshengzu

2. Foot acupuncture: Stiff neck, Lumbago, Kidney, Waist and leg, Ischium1, Ischium 2

IV-4 Eczema 湿疹 Shizhen

- **Differentiation**

1. Acute
It is characterized by a rapid onset of erythema. The clusters and flakes may break by scratching, and it may turn into severe itching sensation, red tongue with sticky coating, and rapid slippery pulse.

2. Chronic
After repeated attacking eczema for a long time, it may be caused blood deficiency. The manifestations are roughness of skin, red tongue with less coating, and rapid thready pulse.

- **Treatment**

1. Foot meridian acupuncture: SP-2 (Dadu 大都)
2. Foot acupuncture: Lung, Tonsil

3. Foot massage: Parathyroid gland, Lung, Adrenal gland, Kidney, Ureter, Urinary bladder, Coeliac plexus, Spleen

IV-5 Erysipelas 丹毒 Dandu

This is an acute contact infection skin disease with red skin lesion.

- **Treatment**
1. Foot acupuncture: Lung
2. Foot massage: Parathyroid gland, Adrenal gland, Kidney, Urinary bladder

IV-6 Furuncle and carbuncle 疖和痈 Jieheyong

The carbuncle is commonly seen in aged people and patients with diabetes mellitus. This is a pyogenic infection of multiple neighboring hair follicles and sebaceous glands or a confluence of several furuncles.

The furuncle occurs on the head, face, hand and foot. It is characterized by chills, fever, thirst, constipation, dark urine.

- **Treatment**
1. Foot meridian acupuncture:
GB-44 (Zuqiaoyin 足窍阴), BL-65 (Shugu 束谷)
2. Foot massage: Reproductive gland, Lymph nodes (upper body), Lymph nodes (abdomen, Adrenal gland

IV-7 Hemorrhoids 痔疮 Zhichuang

It refers to swollen or small pieces of muscle exposed on the anus internally or externally.

- **Differentiation**
1. Internal Hemorrhoids

Damp-Heat Retention:
It involves pain in the anus, and small soft swollen veins in fresh red or purplish green color. The manifestations are feverish sensation in the anus, constipation, red tongue, and rapid pulse.

Qi Deficiency:
The manifestation, pallor complexion, shortness of breath, poor appetite, no energy, prolapse of

swollen veins, pale tongue, and weak thready pulse.

2. External Hemorrhoids
The manifestations are visible swollen veins with big size and hard in nature. It may be caused by long sitting, long standing and anus friction which does not involve bleeding.

- **Treatment**

1. Foot meridian acupuncture:
SP-5 (Shangqiu 商丘), Liv-3 (Taichong 太冲), GB-43 (Xiaxi 侠溪), SP-4 (Gongsun 公孙), KI-6 (Zhaohai 照海), BL-64 (Jinggu 京骨), BL-65 (Shugu 束谷)
2. Foot massage: Anus, Rectum, Anus and Rectum, Sacrum, small intestine, Colon (transverse)

IV-8 prostate gland disease
前列腺炎病 **Qianliexianyanbing**

Hyperplasia of the prostate gland and prostatitis are two major diseases of this gland. Patients with hyperplasia of the prostate gland may suffer from dysuria, frequent urination at night, incomplete urination, and retention of urine which is accompanied by weakness of limbs.

- **Treatment**

1. Foot meridian acupuncture:

BL-67 (Zhiyin 至阴), KI-1 (Yongquan 涌泉), KI-4 (Dazhong 大钟), KI-5 (Shuiquan 水泉), KI-6 (Zhaohai 照海), Liv-1 (Dadun 大敦), Liv-2 (Xingjian 行间), Liv-3 (Taichong 太冲), Liv-4 (Zhongfeng 中风), EX ((Quchi 曲池)

2. Foot acupuncature: Spleen, Kidney, Bladder, Bed-wetting

3. Foot massage: Prostate gland, Ureter, Kidney, Adrenal gland, Urethra, Urinary bladder, Lymph nodes (abdomen), Sacrum

IV-9 Urticaria 荨麻疹 Xunmazhen

It is abrupt onset with itching flat-topped wheals of various size on the skin. In TCM, it calls Wind Wheal.

- **Differentiation**

1. Wind Heat

The manifestations are red rashes, severe itching, rapid pulse.

2. Wind Damp
The manifestations are Light red or white rashes superficial and rapid pulse.

3. Accumulation of Heat in the Stomach and Intestine
The manifestations are, red rashes, abdominal pain, constipation, diarrhea, thin yellow tongue coating, and rapid pulse.

- **Treatment**

1. Foot meridian acupuncture:
KI-1 (Yongquan 涌泉), ST-44 (Neiting 内庭), Liv-2 (Xingjian 行间), ST-41 (Jiexi 解溪), LI-4 (Hegu 合谷), SJ-4 (Yangchi 阳池) on hand.

2. Foot acupuncture: Lung, Ischium
3. Foot massage: Lung, Parathyroid gland, Kidney, Colon (transverse), Liver, Gallbladder, Adrenal gland, Lymph nodes (upper body, chest, abdomen)

V. Diseases of Eye, Ear, Nose, and Throat and Oral Cavity

V-1 Aphtha 口疮 Kouchuang

This is the oral cavity with yellowish white ulcers the size of a pea on the buccal mucosa. It is divided into excessive and deficient types.

1. Deficient type
Ulcers are caused by the upward flaming of deficient fire.

2. Excessive type
Ulcers are caused by overeating greasy food, alcohol, accumulation of heat in Spleen and Stomach, and transformation of heat pathogens to fire attacking the oral cavity along the meridian. They are yellowish white ulcers on lips, tongue, and buccal mucosa in a round or elliptic shape, the size of a pea, surrounded by a fresh red border.

- **Treatment**
  1. Foot meridian acupuncture: ST-45 (Lidui 厉兑)
  2. Foot acupuncture: Head and face, Heart, Kidney

3. Foot massage: Palate, Lower jaw, Lymph nodes (upper body), Frontal sinus, Trigeminal nerve

V-2 Aphonia 失音 Shiyin

This is a disease of the oral cavity with yellowish white ulcers the size of a pea on the buccal mucosa.

- **Differentiation**

1. Excess Type

(1) Wind-Cold:

The sudden hoarseness of voice is accompanied by difficult cough, fullness in the chest, stuffy nose, chills, fever, headache, with thin white tongue coating and superficial pulse.

(2) Phlegm-Heat:

The sudden low voice or husky voice is accompanied by cough, yellow sputum, sore throat, dry nose, fever, thirst, thin yellow tongue coating and rapid superficial pulse.

(3) Qi Stagnation:

The sudden aphonia that is often induced by emotional upset such as sorrow, grief, depression or anger appears paroxysmal. It is accompanied by restlessness, irritability, suffocating sensation in the chest, or a foreign body sensation in the throat, thin yellow tongue coating and thready pulse.

2. Deficient Type
The progressive aphonia is accompanied by dry throat, thirst, tidal fever, night sweating, dry cough, palpitation, dizziness, tinnitus, red tongue with less coating, and thin rapid pulse.

- **Treatment**
1. Foot meridian acupuncture:
ST-45 (Lidui 厉兑)
2. Foot acupuncture: Head and face, Heart, Kidney
3. Foot massage: Throat, Trachea, Vocal cord, Tonsil, Lymph nodes, Lymph nodes (abdomen), Neck

V-3 Myopia 近视 Jinshi

It is characterized in that the eyes can see near objects but not distant.

- **Differentiation**

It is clear for near objects but blurred vision for distant which may be accompanied by tinnitus, insomnia, dizziness, pale tongue, and weak thready pulse.

- **Treatment**

1. Foot meridian acupuncture:
ST-44 (Neiting 内庭), GB-41 (Zulinqi 足临泣), GB-42 (Diwuhui 地五会), GB-43 (Xiaxi 侠溪), GB-44 (Zuqiaoyin 足窍阴), BL-60 (Kunlun 昆仑), BL-64 (Jinggu 京骨)

2. Foot acupuncture: Head and face, Liver, Kidney

3. Foot massage: Eye, Frontal sinus, Parathyroid gland, Kidney, Adrenal gland, Ureter, Urinary bladder, Liver

V-4 Nasal bleeding 鼻出血 Bichuxie

This is a condition caused by trauma, inflammation, polyp or tumor of nose

- **Treatment**

1. Foot meridian acupuncture:

BL-60 (Kunlun 昆仑), ST-45 (Lidui 厉兑), BL-62 (Shenmai 申脉), BL-64 (Jinggu 京骨), BL-66 (Zutonggu 足通谷), BL-67 (Zhiyin 至阴), KI-1 (Yongquan 涌泉), KI-3 (Taixi 太溪), Liv-2 (Xingjian 行间)
2. Foot acupuncture: Head and face, Lung
3. Foot massage: Frontal sinus, Nose, Parathyroid gland, Lymph nodes (upper body, chest, abdomen)

V-5 Optic atrophy 视神经萎缩 Shishenjingweisuo

This is a chronic eye disorder by gradual degeneration of vision.

- **Differentiation**

1. Liver and Kidney Deficiency
The manifestations are dizziness, tinnitus, dryness of the eye, blurred vision, lower back pain, red tongue with scanty coating, weak pulse.

2. Qi and Blood Deficiency

The manifestations are lassitude, loose stools, blurred vision, weakness of breath, pale tongue with thin coating, weak thready pulse.

- **Treatment**

1. Foot meridian acupuncture:

GB-41 (Zulinqi 足临泣), Liv-2 (Xingjian 行间）, KI-6 (Zhaohai 照海), BL-67 (Zhiyin 至阴)

2. Foot acupuncture: Head and face, Liver, Kidney

3. Foot massage: Eye, Kidney, Adrenal gland, Ureter, Urinary bladder, Head (brain), Brain stem, Cerebellum, Lymph nodes (upper body), Lymph nodes (abdomen), Liver

V-6 Presbyopia 老花眼 Laohuayan

This is a gradual impairment of vision of old age with blurred vision, heaviness of eyelids.

- **Treatment**

1. Foot meridian acupuncture:

ST-45 (Lidui 厉兑), BL-65 (Shugu 束谷), GB-41 (Zulinqi 足临泣), GB-42 (Diwuhui 地五会), GB-44 (Zuqiaoyin 足窍阴), BL-62 (Shenmai 申脉), BL-67

(Zhiyin 至阴), KI-6 (Zhaohai 照海), Liv-2 (Xingjian 行间), Liv-3 (Taichong 太冲)

2. Foot acupuncture: Head and face, Liver, Kidney

3. Foot massage: Eye, Shoulder, Neck, Liver, Kidney, Reproductive gland

V-7 Red eyes 红眼睛 Hongyanjing

This red eye is an acute with redness, swelling, pain watery or dry.

- **Treatment**

  1. Foot meridian acupuncture:

  ST-44 (Neiting 内庭), GB-41 (Zulinqi 足临泣), GB-42 (Diwuhui)地五会, GB-43 (Xiaxi 侠溪), GB-44 (Zuqiaoyin足窍阴), BL-60 (Kunlun 昆仑), BL-62 (Shenmai 申脉), BL-64 (Jinggu 京骨), BL-65 (Shugu 束谷), BL-66 (Zutonggu 足通谷), BL-67 (Zhiyin 至阴), KI-6 (Zhaohai 照海), Liv-2 (Xingjian 行间), Liv-3 (Taichong 太冲)

  2. Foot acupuncture: Head and face, Liver, Kidney

3. Foot massage: Eye, Frontal sinus, Head, Kidney, Liver, Lymph nodes (upper body), Lymph nodes (abdomen)

V-8 Stye (Hordeolum) 大麦 (麦粒肿) Damai (mailizhong)

It is characterized by itching and painful nodule which is the size of a grain of wheat on the eyelid.
It refers to the inflammatory furuncle of the sebaceous gland of the eyelid, and often occurs among young people.

- **Differentiation**
The manifestations are itching, redness, pain, yellow greasy tongue coating, and soft rapid pulse. It may be caused Damp-Heat from Spleen and Stomach, and accompanies fever, headache, thin tongue coating, rapid pulse.

- **Treatment**
1. Foot meridian acupuncture:
ST-44(Neiting 内庭), GB-41 (Zulinqi 足临泣), GB-42 (Diwuhui 地五会), GB-43 (Xiaxi 侠溪), GB-44 (Zuqiaoyin 足窍阴), BL-62 (Shenmai 申脉), BL-64

(Jinggu 京骨), BL-65 (Shugu 束谷), BL-67 (Zhiyin 至阴), KI-6 (Zhaohai 照海), Liv-2 (Xingjian 行间), Liv-3 (Taichong 太冲)

2. Foot acupuncture: Head and face, Liver, Kidney

3. Foot massage: Eye, Parathyroid gland, Lymph nodes (upper body), Lymph nodes (abdomen), Kidney, Liver

V-9 Sinusitis 鼻窦炎 Bidouyan

This disease is caused by an allergy to fur, fibers, pollen, dust, chemicals. It is characterized by sneezing, running nose, nasal obstruction.

Foot therapy produces 90 percent cure rate.

- **Treatment**
  1. Foot meridian acupuncture:
  BL-64 (Jinggu 京骨)
  2. Foot acupuncture: Head and face, Lung
  3. Foot massage:
  *Allergic rhinitis: Nose, throat and trachea, lung, pituitary gland, adrenal gland, lymph nodes.

*Sinusitis: Nose, Parathyroid gland, Lymph nodes (upper body), Lymph nodes (abdomen), frontal sinus

V-10 Sore Throat 咽喉肿 Yanhouzhongtong

It can be caused by external pathogens or internal injury.
It is similar to tonsillitis.

- ## Differentiation

1. Excess Heat
This is abrupt onset with fever, headache, pain in the throat, constipation, thirst, red tongue with thin yellow coating, superficial rapid pulse.

2. Deficient Heat
Gradual onset without fever, dry throat, feverish sensation in palms and soles, red uncoated tongue, and rapid thready pulse.

- ## Treatment
1. Foot meridian acupuncture:
(Sore throat caused by external pathogens)

ST-44 (Neiting 内庭), ST-42 (Chongyang 冲阳), ST-45 (Lidui 厉兑), GB-41 (Zulinqi 足临泣)

(Sore throat caused by internal injury)
KI-1 (Yongquan 涌泉), KI-3 (Taixi 太溪), KI-6 (Zhaohai 照海), Liv-3 (Taichong 太冲)
2. Foot acupuncture:
Tonsil1, Tonsil 2, Head and face, Heart, Kidney
3. Foot massage: Neck, Tonsil, Throat, Ear, Chest, Lymph nodes (upper body), Kidney, Adrenal gland, Urinary bladder

V-11 Tinnitus and Deafness 耳鸣 耳聋 Erming Erlong

Tinnitus is characterized by continuous ringing of the ear, and Deafness refers to loss of hearing and low degree of hearing.

- **Differentiation**

1. Excess of Liver and Gallbladder
Tinnitus: It is continuous ringing in the ear and there is no relieving.
Deafness: Sudden deafness.

The manifestations are irritability, heavy sensation of the head, bitter taste in mouth, red tongue with yellow coating rapid wiry pulse.

2. Deficiency of Kidney Essence
Tinnitus: It is intermittent ringing, and it becomes aggravated after stress and strain, but it is alleviated by pressure.
Deafness: It is gradually intensified deafness.
The manifestations are dizziness, lassitude, low back pain, insomnia, red tongue with little coating, and weak thready pulse.

- **Treatment**

1. Foot meridian acupuncture:
ST-44 (Neiting 内庭), GB-41 (Zulinqi 足临泣), GB-42 (Diwuhui 地五会), GB-43 (Xiaxi 侠溪), GB-44 (Zuqiaoyin 足窍阴), BL-62 (Shenmai 申脉), BL-63 (Jinmen 金门), BL-65 (Shugu 束谷), KI-3 (Taixi 太溪)
2. Foot acupuncture: Head and face, Kidney, Vertigo
3. Foot massage: Ear, Labyrinth, Head, Lymph nodes (upper body), Lymph nodes (abdomen), Parathyroid gland

V-12 Toothache 齿痛 Chitong

- **Differentiation**

1. Wind-Heat
Toothache follows swelling, pain, preference for cold food, fever, constipation, red tongue with white coating, and rapid pulse.

2. Kidney Deficiency
Toothache follows intermittent pain, loose teeth, red tongue, and rapid thready pulse.

- **Treatment**

1. Foot meridian acupuncture:
ST-42 (Chongyang 冲阳), ST-44 (Neiting 内庭), ST-45 (Lidui 厉兑), GB-41 (Zulinqi 足临泣), BL-60 (Kunlun 昆仑), KI-3 (Taixi 太溪), EX (Waihuaiqian Jiaomai), EX (Nuxi), EX (Bafeng 八风)
2. Foot acupuncture:
Head and face, Toothache 1, Toothache 2
3. Foot massage: Neck, Palate, Low jaw, Stomach, Liver, Small intestine, Lymph nodes (upper body)

V-13 Trigeminal Neuralgia 三叉神经痛 Sanchashenjingtong

Trigeminal nerves are divided into three branches, which are supraorbital branch, maxillary branch and mandibular branch.

- **Differentiation**
It is manifested by sudden onset of facial pain, occurs in transient paroxysms, and just like being cutting, burning, and needling, which lasts in a few seconds or few minutes, and several times a day. It is accompanied by local spasm, lacrimation, and salivation.

- **Treatment**
1. Foot meridian acupuncture:
ST-45 (Lidui 厉兑), ST-41 (Jiexi 解溪), ST-42 (Chongyang 冲阳), GB-43 (Xiaxi 侠溪), KI-3 (Taixi 太溪), Liv-2 (Xingjian 行间)
2. Foot acupuncture: Face, Liver, Stomach
3. Foot massage: Head, Frontal sinus, Liver, Stomach, Kidney, Eye, Ear, Palate, Lower jaw

References 参考文献

1. Zhou Qinghui, Wrist-Ankle Acupuncture, 2002.

2. Wang Lingline, Diagram of Chinese Acupoints, 2005

2. Ji Qingshan, Foot Therapy for Common Diseases, 2001

3. Musculoskeletal Key.

4. E. Akimoto, Hand and Foot point.

5. Foot reflective zones chart.

6. Sumiko Knudsen, Body Acupuncture Clinical Treatment

7. Sumiko Knudsen, Acupuncture Meridians and Points

Other library of Traditional Chinese Medicine by Sumiko Knudsen

1. Acupuncture for Weight Loss
2. Akupunkture til Vægttab
3. Acupuncture Meridians and Points
4. Akupunktur Meridianer og Punkter
5. Ear Acupuncture
6. Øre Akupunktur
7. Body Acupuncture, Clinical Treatment
8. Krop Akupunktur, Klinisk Behandling
9. Acupuncture and Moxibustion
10. Akupunktur og Moxibustion
11. Scalp Acupuncture
12. Hovedbundsakupunktur
13. Hand Acupuncture Clinical Treatment
14. Hånd Akupunktur Klinisk Behandling
15. Fod Akupunktur Klinisk Behandling